Pro-drugs as Novel Drug Delivery Systems

Pro-drugs as Novel Drug Delivery Systems

T. Higuchi and **V. Stella,** *Editors*

A symposium sponsored by
the Division of Medicinal
Chemistry at the 168th
Meeting of the American
Chemical Society,
Atlantic City, N.J.,
September 10, 1974.

ACS SYMPOSIUM SERIES **14**

AMERICAN CHEMICAL SOCIETY

WASHINGTON, D. C.   1975

Library of Congress CIP Data

Pro-drugs as novel drug delivery systems.
  (ACS symposium series; 14)

  Includes bibliographies and index.

  1. Chemistry, Medical and pharmaceutical—Congresses.
2. Drug metabolism—Congresses.
  I. Higuchi, Takeru, 1918-   II. Stella, V., 1946-
III. American Chemical Society. Division of Medicinal
Chemistry.   IV. American Chemical Society.   V. Title.
VI. Series: American Chemical Society. ACS symposium
series; 14.

RS421.S92 1974   615'.7   75-11721
ISBN 0-8412-0291-5   ACSMC8 14 1–245

6100441820

ACS Symposium Series

Robert F. Gould, *Series Editor*

FOREWORD

The ACS Symposium Series was founded in 1974 to provide
a medium for publishing symposia quickly in book form. The
format of the Series parallels that of its predecessor, Advances
in Chemistry Series, except that in order to save time the
papers are not typeset but are reproduced as they are sub-
mitted by the authors in camera-ready form. As a further
means of saving time, the papers are not edited or reviewed
except by the symposium chairman, who becomes editor of
the book. Papers published in the ACS Symposium Series
are original contributions not published elsewhere in whole or
major part and include reports of research as well as reviews
since symposia may embrace both types of presentation.

CONTENTS

vii

PREFACE

This volume contains the papers presented during the Symposium on Pro-drugs held at Atlantic City, September 10, 1974 under the sponsorship of the Division of Medicinal Chemistry. No serious effort was made in organizing the program to provide a comprehensive treatment of the subject matter. Rather it was hoped that the material presented would stimulate greater interest in this chemical approach to the problem of drug delivery.

A short review of the subject sets forth some of the basic underlying concepts and approaches. Applications of the pro-drug principle to an array of antibiotics are then discussed. The remainder of the volume details chemical and biological studies on pro-drug candidates developed in our own laboratories.

We apologize for the limited coverage of the subject matter contained in this book. This was caused more by necessity than by choice. At the time the program was formulated we were forced to depend largely on projects completed or being carried out in our several facilities or in those of our collaborators. This was in large part due to the sensitive nature of pro-drug research programs in established drug houses and their reluctance to publicize their early efforts in the field. In any case, the examples have been selected to illustrate the real utility of this approach.

I would like to take this opportunity to thank all those who took part in the program and Naida Jimenez and her able secretarial assistants for their help in preparing the manuscript.

University of Kansas   TAKERU HIGUCHI
Lawrence, Kans.
March 11, 1975

Pro-drugs: An Overview and Definition

V. STELLA

University of Kansas, Department of Pharmaceutical Chemistry, Lawrence, Kans. 66044

Historically the term pro-drug was first introduced by Albert (1,2) who used the word "pro-drug" or "pro-agent" to describe compounds which undergo biotransformation prior to exhibiting their pharmacological effects. Albert suggested that this concept could be used for many different purposes. For example, in his book "Selective Toxicity" (2) he mentions that "as a means of introducing selectivity into toxicity, the principle of latent activity has endless possibilities." Albert himself points out that the pro-drug approach is not new. Methenamine (I) and aspirin (II), both synthesized in the late nineteenth century, are examples of bioreversible derivatives of

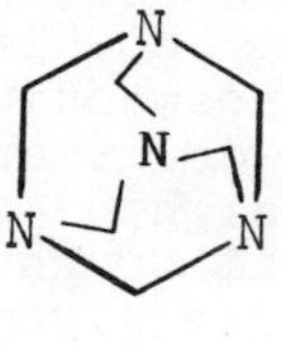

(I) 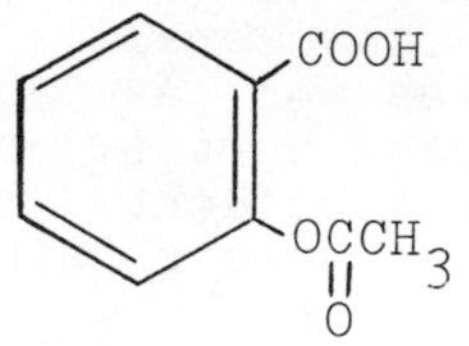   (II)

formaldehyde and salicylic acid respectively. Use of salicylic acid as an analgesic and anti-inflammatory agent was somewhat limited by its corrosiveness which was in part overcome with the use of II. Formaldehyde, although a useful topical antiseptic, could not be used orally as a urinary tract antiseptic until it was converted to I and formulated in an enteric coated tablet.

The chemical modification of drugs to overcome pharmaceutical problems has also been termed "drug

latentiation." The term was first used by Harper
(3,4) following the suggestion of Dr. L. Golberg.
Harper defined drug latentiation "as the chemical
modification of a biologically active compound to form
a new compound which upon in vivo enzymatic attack
will liberate the parent compound. The chemical al-
terations of the parent compound are such that the
change in physicochemical properties will affect the
absorption, distribution and enzymatic metabolism."
Kupchan et al. (5), in attempting to utilize the pro-
drug or drug latentiation approach for solving various
problems, extended the definition of drug latentiation
to include nonenzymatic regeneration of the parent
compound. Regeneration takes place as a consequence
of hydrolytic, dissociative and other reactions not
necessarily enzyme mediated.
    The terms pro-drugs, latentiated drugs and bio-
reversible derivatives have been used interchangeably.
Sinkula and Yalkowsky in their review (6) state, "by
inference, latentiation implies a time lag element or
time component involved in regenerating the bioactive
parent molecule in vivo . . . . the term pro-drug is
general in that it includes latentiated drug derivatives as well as those substances which are converted
after administration to the actual substance which
combines with receptors."
    The term pro-drug is a catchy, generic term for
agents which undergo biotransformation prior to exhibiting their pharmacological actions and will be
used in this manuscript to describe both specifically
designed bioreversible derivatives of a troublesome
compound as well as "accidents" or retrospective pro-
drugs. As Albert (2) states, many pro-drugs are the
result of "accidents" rather than foresighted attempts
to overcome some physiological, physical or psychological barrier. For example, anthracene glycosides
exhibit their laxative action through their aglycone
while codeine may exert its action due to the formation of morphine (2).
    The utilization of the pro-drug approach has been
growing since scientists began to realize that problems such as lack of solubility, poor bioavailability
due to polarity or "first pass" effect, or lack of
chemical stability could be overcome by preparing
chemically altered temporary transport forms of the
drug (see III). Once the barrier to the use of the
parent compound has been overcome, these temporary
transport forms can be converted to the parent compound. This releases the transport moiety "C," which

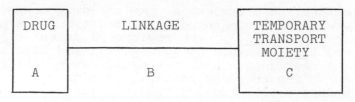

DRUG	LINKAGE	TEMPORARY TRANSPORT MOIETY
A	B	C

(III)

obviously has to be nontoxic, so that the parent drug is free to exert its pharmacological activity.

Is a salt or a complex of a drug a pro-drug? The question of defining drug derivatives as pro-drugs can be quite controversial. Linkage "B" is normally thought of as a covalent bond, e.g., an ester linkage, a phosphate ester linkage, etc. However, historically such products as benzathine penicillin have been viewed as pro-drugs or as examples of drug latentiation (3,4), yet the linkage "B" between the parent compound, penicillin, and the transport moiety, benzathine, is electrostatic. The regeneration of penicillin from benzathine penicillin is simply dissociation of this poorly water soluble salt. A complex or a salt is a chemically defined new substance, i.e., a new thermodynamic entity, just as a modification involving covalent bonding results in a new chemical substance. If the physical and chemical properties of this new substance give it unique qualities capable of overcoming some undesirable barrier to the use of the parent compound and this new substance reverts to the parent compound after overcoming this barrier, then it is the belief of this author that no matter how trivial the chemical modification may be, the new substance is a pro-drug of the parent compound. A number of semantic arguments for and against this definition can be made and reservations about calling the salt of a compound a pro-drug would be readily admitted. However, procaine and benzathine penicillin (7-11), and mafenide acetate (salt not amide) for topical application (12-14) are examples of specific salt forms of a parent compound which impart unique and important qualities to the stable, prolonged, and efficient release characteristics of the parent compound. Similarly, the discussion later by Dr. Repta of the water soluble gentisate complex of hexamethylmelamine will demonstrate the uniqueness of this combination over the parent compound, thus qualifying the complex as a pro-drug of hexamethylmelamine.

Reviews and overviews of the pro-drug concept are numerous. Apart from the classic reviews of Harper (3,4) and Albert (1,2), the reviews of Ariens (15-18), Bundgaard (19), Sinkula et al. (6,20), and Stella (21) should be mentioned. Each review offers a different approach to the pro-drug concept, even though obvious overlap does exist. Notari (22), in his recent thesis on pharmacokinetics and molecular modification, touches lightly on the pharmacokinetic implications of the pro-drug approach, an area of study which deserves much more attention.

Rationale for the Use of Pro-Drugs

The awareness that a drug can only exert a desired pharmacological effect if it reaches its site of action has recently been reemphasized by the resurgence and growth of pharmacokinetics which is the study of the time course of absorption, distribution, metabolism and excretion of drugs. The concentration versus time profile of a drug, its metabolite in various tissues and organs, and the time profile of the corresponding pharmacological response has been a particularly exciting and fruitful area in current pharmacokinetic research (23-25). The awareness that the onset, intensity and duration of drug action are greatly affected by the physical and chemical properties of the drug has promoted the emergence of various theoretical and predictive models for drug design and evaluation (26-28).

Ariens et al. (29) point out that drug action involves three major phases: the pharmaceutical phase, the pharmacokinetic phase, and the pharmacodynamic phase. The pharmacodynamic phase represents the drug-receptor interaction or biological availability of the drug. Scheme I shows a simplified pharmacokinetic model for a typical drug entity and demonstrates that before a drug-receptor interaction can occur the drug must reach the target organ in which the drug receptor is located. A number of barriers may limit a drug's ability to reach a desired target organ and the subsequent receptor site and these barriers can be of pharmacokinetic origin. To reach an effective and desired concentration of drug at the target organ requires not only the drug to be efficiently absorbed ($f \sim 1$ and k_1 either large relative to other rate constants or controlled) but it also ideally requires that the amount of drug in the rest of the body be minimized to prevent toxicity. The pathway shown by the broken line and rate constants k'_1 and k'_2 would

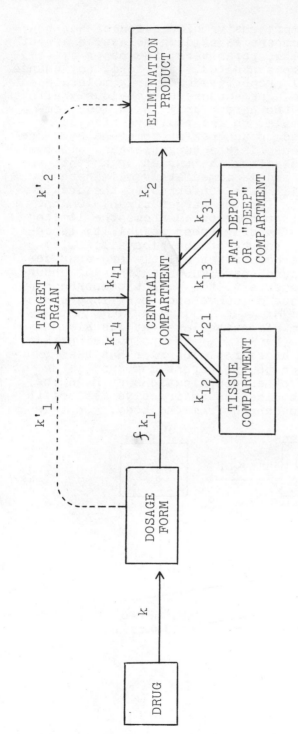

Scheme I

where k_i = rate constants defining the transport of a drug between various components

k_2 = $k_{excretion}$ + $k_{metabolism}$ + k_{other}

f = fraction of dose absorbed

be ideal. For a comprehensive discussion of how the
physical chemical properties of drug molecules affect
various pharmacokinetic parameters, the paper by
Notari (22) should be consulted. A priori, any change
in physical chemical properties of a drug molecule due
to its conversion to a pro-drug could obviously affect
the time profile of the parent drug in various com-
partments. For example, on the positive side, a pro-
drug may be converted to the parent compound by a specific enzyme found only in the target organ. If the
parent compound passes from the target organ into the
central compartment and is immediately eliminated,
then the pro-drug will have conferred to the drug a
degree of specificity for the target organ. On the
other hand, if in attempting to overcome the limited
aqueous solubility of a drug (poor solubility is defined as the primary source of the bioavailability
problem) a well absorbed, water soluble pro-drug derivative is synthesized, care must be taken to ensure
that the pro-drug reverts to the parent compound
(Scheme II). The rate of conversion must insure a
buildup in concentration of the parent drug to a level above its minimum effective level at its site of
action, i.e., $k_4 \gg (k_3 + k_2)$, the point being that
once the particular undesirable barrier has been overcome, rapid reversion to the parent compound is desirable to minimize other complications such as the
pro-drug being metabolized to an inactive metabolite
or being excreted unchanged from the body. On this

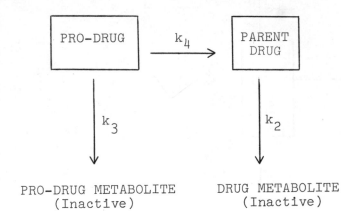

Scheme II

point, Albert (2) commented that "although a detailed
knowledge of permeability and enzymes can assist a
skillful designer in finding useful pro-agents, he
will have in mind an organism's normal reaction of a
foreign substance is to burn it up for food."

Barriers of nonpharmacokinetic and nonpharmaco-
dynamic origin may also play a major role in preventing a drug from reaching a desired target organ.
Referring to Scheme I, it is obvious that there are
other barriers (represented by the rate constant k)
inhibiting the drug's ability to reach the dosage form
stage. The rejection of a product can be due to pa-
thological limitations such as toxicity and high in-
cidences of side effects, teratogenicity, etc. Pharmaceutical limitations include such factors as the
chemical instability of the compound or formulation
difficulties. Common psychological limitations can be
traced to the unpleasant taste of a drug, pain at an
injection site, or cosmetic damage to the patient.
Economic barriers which are also important are often
overlooked. In the economic structure of our society,
a drug must have the potential to make economic gains
for its promotor or it will not reach the market
place. Just as pro-drugs can be used to overcome
pharmacokinetic barriers, pro-drugs have been used to
overcome nonpharmacokinetic barriers. An unpatented,
pharmacologically active drug with some physico-chem-
ical properties limiting its usefulness may not be of
interest to a large company. If, however, the barrier
to the drug's use is successfully removed by bioreversible chemical modification and the modification is
patentable, the product may then have economic potential.

The design of efficient, stable, safe, patient
acceptable and esthetically pleasing way to deliver
a drug to its site of action while overcoming various
physical, chemical and social barriers is certainly an
area where the utilization of the pro-drug approach
holds great potential. Figure 1 shows the types of
barriers that have limited the successful screening
and/or full development of suspected pharmacologically
active agents and for which the pro-drug approach has
proven to be successful in overcoming.

Applications of the Pro-drug Approach

It is not the objective of this overview to discuss every possible example where the pro-drug concept
was used to overcome a problem. That would be an arduous task. What will be presented will be a brief

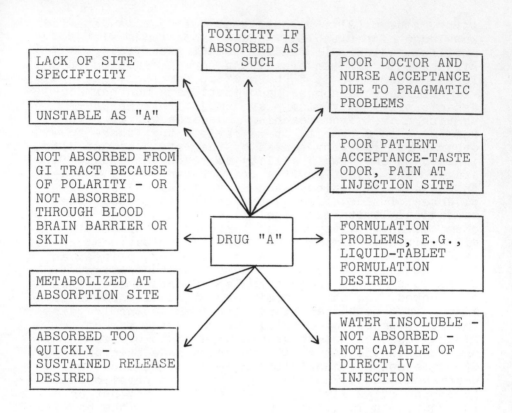

Figure 1

listing and discussion of some of the more classic
examples as well as some recent developments. Hope-
fully, this approach will encourage application of the
pro-drug concept to current research and problem solving by others.
     The pro-drug approach has apparently led to a
great deal of success in overcoming specific problems
associated with certain drug molecules. Many of the
examples that will be given in this review are what
may be called foresighted pro-drugs, i.e., cases where
the scientist has, through the use of the knowledge of
factors affecting drug absorption, distribution, metabolism and excretion, designed and synthesized pro-
drugs with the specific view to overcome some problem
associated with the parent compound. At the same
time, there are many examples of "accidental" pro-
drugs which, in retrospect, have been found to be very
useful and significantly superior to the parent com-

pound. When the rationale for the design or use of a particular pro-drug is discussed, it should be stated that the current application of the pro-drug may not have been the reason for synthesizing the pro-drug in the first place.

Use of Pro-Drugs in Overcoming Absorption Problems

To state that the pro-drug approach has been used to overcome absorption problems is rather meaningless unless the particular absorption barrier is defined. For example, a drug may be poorly absorbed from the gastrointestinal (GI) tract, into the central nervous system (CNS), into the eye or through the skin, etc., because the drug is too polar. Quaternary ammonium compounds and other highly polar chemicals are not well absorbed through these barriers because the barriers are lipoidal in nature. The qualifying statement should be made that some highly polar molecules such as vitamins, amino acids and carbohydrates are absorbed through these barriers but are absorbed by active transport. A drug may be poorly absorbed from the GI tract because of the very water insoluble characteristics of the drug. The rate determining step to absorption may become the dissolution rate of the drug. Also, a drug may apparently be poorly absorbed into general circulation as a result of the so-called "first pass" effect (30-34). The "first pass" effect results from the loss of the drug due to metabolism of the drug in the GI mucosa or liver in its initial passage through these organs.

Understanding the problem drugs would be an easy task if they could be partitioned into neat categories. Invariably, poor absorption of a drug cannot be attributed to any single factor.

To Facilitate Passage Through Lipid Membranes of Drugs with Poor Lipid Solubility.

Catecholamines. Chemical modification to increase lipid solubility and to facilitate the absorption of pharmacologically active catecholamines from the GI tract and through the blood brain barrier (BBB) has led to a great deal of study. Moderate success has been achieved to date.

Deficiencies of brain dopamine (IV) resulting from degeneration of the substantia nigra seem to be associated with a number of symptoms of Parkinson's disease (35-40). Therefore, attempts have been made to raise the brain levels of dopamine in patients

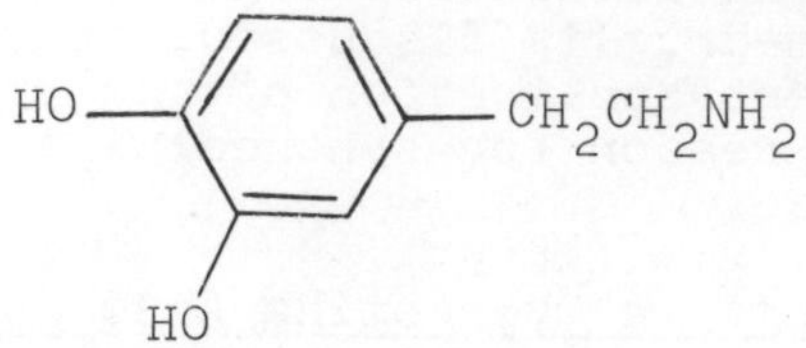

HO—⟨ring⟩—CH₂CH₂NH₂ with HO substituent below

$$HO-\underset{HO}{\bigcirc}-CH_2CH_2NH_2$$

(IV)

suffering from Parkinson's disease. It has been
stated that dopamine itself cannot be used because it
is incapable of being absorbed across the BBB, a fact
primarily attributed to dopamine's high polarity and
highly ionized state at physiological pH. A precursor
or a pro-drug of dopamine, L-Dopa (V) or L-3,4-dihy-
droxyphenylalanine, has repeatedly been found to be
effective in the treatment of Parkinson's disease
(41-50). L-Dopa is absorbed from the GI tract and

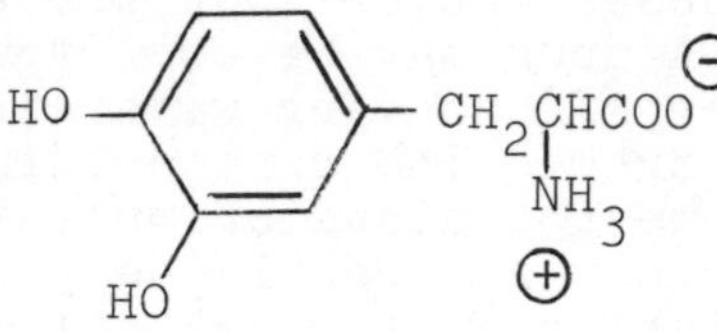

$$HO-\underset{HO}{\bigcirc}-CH_2\underset{\overset{\mid}{NH_3^{\oplus}}}{CH}COO^{\ominus}$$

(V)

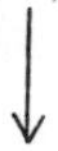

$\downarrow$ DOPA DECARBOXYLASE

DOPAMINE

into the CNS through the active transport mechanism
for amino acids (51-52). In the CNS, Dopa decarboxylase can convert L-Dopa to the desired dopamine. It
has been assumed that the poor absorption of dopamine
is due to its polarity and highly ionized state. However, rapid enzymatic metabolism of catechol molecules
via conjugation mechanisms such as sulfation, glucuronidation and O-methylation contribute heavily to
the rapid loss of dopamine if dopamine is administered
orally, i.e., dopamine given orally probably never
reaches the BBB. Even with L-Dopa, approximately only
20% of an orally administered dose reaches general
circulation as L-Dopa since it can be rapidly conjugated, decarboxylated, O-methylated and oxidized in
the GI tract and mucosa (53-60). The degree of this
so called "first pass" effect in any given individual

patient is a function of the age, genetic structure, diet, etc. of the individual.

It has been suggested that part of this "first pass" effect might be circumvented by the use of L-Dopa esters (VI) which can be transformed to the

$$HO - \langle \rangle - CH_2\underset{NH_2}{\overset{|}{C}}HCOOR$$

(VI):   R = alkyl substituent

active drug, L-Dopa, following absorption (61). Initially this may seem incongruous because it appears that the ester should have the same absorption problems as dopamine itself, i.e., VI is a primary amine and the catechol groups have not been protected from metabolism. The ionization of phenolic amines including L-Dopa has recently been discussed by Martin (62) and others (63-66). The ionization characteristics of molecules similar to dopamine can be depicted schematically by Schemes III and IV. In these schemes K_1 and K_2 represent the normal macroscopic or observed ionization constants and k_1, k_2, k_{12}, and k_{21} are microscopic ionization constants. If it is assumed that only N〰OH or (00) is absorbed through lipoidal mem-

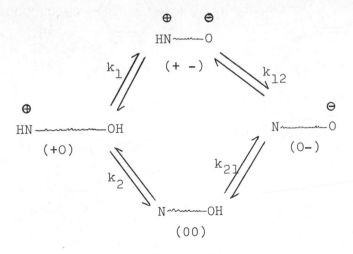

Scheme III

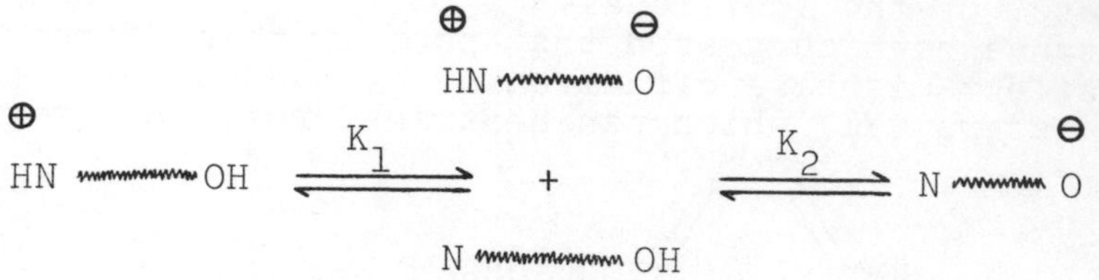

Scheme IV

branes, then the percentage of total drug present at
physiological pH of 7.4 as (00) will be a function of
the various microscopic constants. (For a full discussion of the interrelationships of the microscopic
and macroscopic constants see references 62-66). The
following drugs were subjected to analysis of %(00)
present at physiological pH; tyramine (VII), tyrosine
ethyl ester (VIII), epinephrine (IX), dopamine (IV),
and morphine (X). An estimate of pK_1, pK_2, pk_1, and
pk_2 for a typical L-Dopa ester (VI) was made and approximate %(00) calculated at physiological pH. Table
I gives the pK_1, pK_2, pk_1, pk_2, R(where R is the ratio (+-)/(00) and equals k_1/k_2) and %(00) at physiological pH for these compounds. As is readily apparent from this table little passive absorption from the

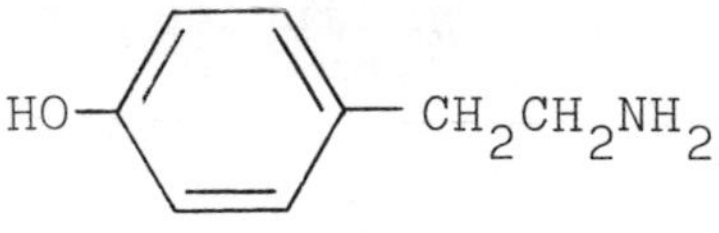

(VII)

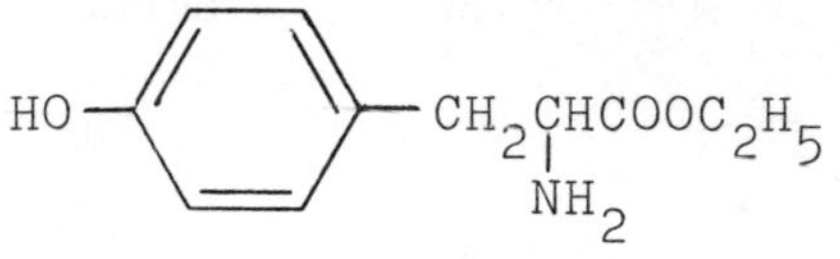

(VIII)

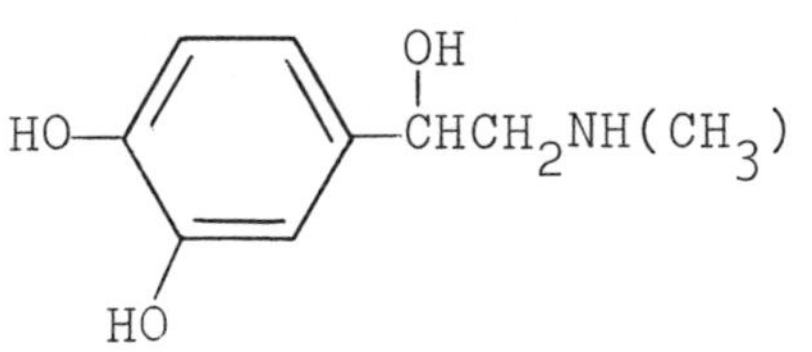

(IX)

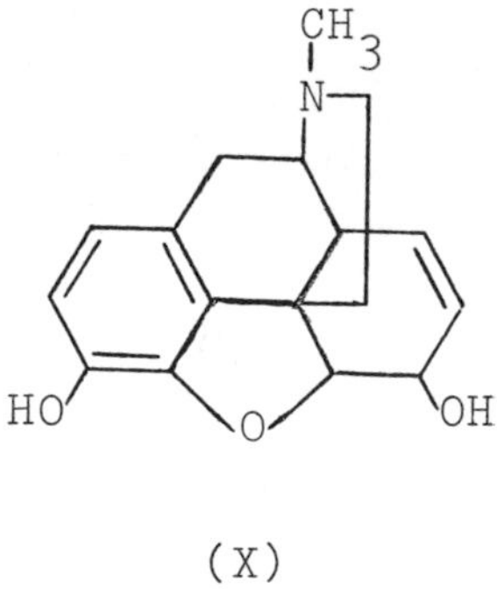

(X)

Table I

Compound	pK_1	pK_2	pk_1	pk_2	R	%(00)
IV	8.87	10.63	8.90	10.06	15	0.21
VI	7.21*	9.44*	8.76*	7.22*	0.03*	60.2*
VII	9.61	10.65	9.70	10.32	4.2	0.12
VIII	7.33	9.80	9.42	7.33	0.008	53.1
IX	8.66	9.95	8.72	9.57	7.1	0.98
X	8.31	9.51	8.87	8.45	0.38	7.98

*Roughly estimated from the data of Martin (62) based on the effect on pK_1, pK_2, pk_1, pk_2 of esterification of the carboxyl group of tyrosine to give tyrosine ethyl ester.

GI tract or through the BBB would be expected for IV, VII or IX unless some compensation for the small fraction of (00) present is made in terms of increased lipophilicity and/or reduced "first pass" metabolism. The rather high fraction of (00) present at physiological pH for VI, VIII and X suggests that these compounds should have little problem penetrating lipoidal membranes, assuming they possess sufficient lipophilicity. Any reduced bioavailability of these compounds can probably be attributed to a "first pass" effect.

Lai et al. (61) have synthesized esters of L-Dopa in an attempt to overcome the "first pass" metabolism of L-Dopa while Anden et al. (67) have prepared the methyl ester of tyrosine to help absorption and prevent decarboxylation.

Pinder suggested 0,0-diacetyl-(XI), 0,0-di(trimethylsilyl)dopamine (XII) as useful pro-drugs of dopamine capable of penetrating the BBB (68). If it is assumed that pk_2, the microscopic ionization constant for the amino group of dopamine, is unaffected by acylation or silyation of the hydroxy groups, %(00) is calculated to be 0.22, i.e., acylation of the hydroxy groups does little to improve the fraction of neutral species present at physiological pH. What acylation may do is protect the hydroxy groups from being conjugated and increase the lipophilicity of the molecule. Pinder based his suggestions on the results

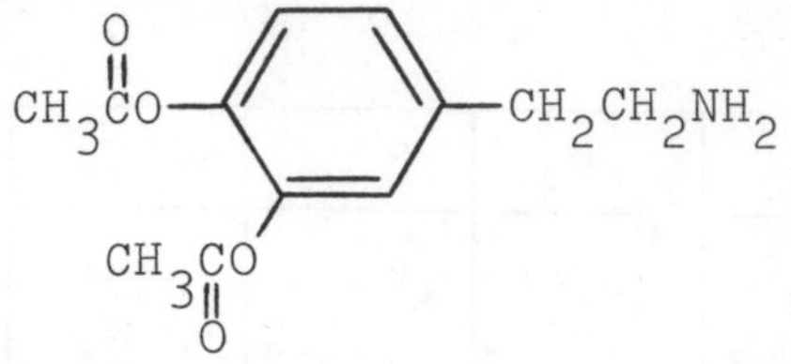

(XI)

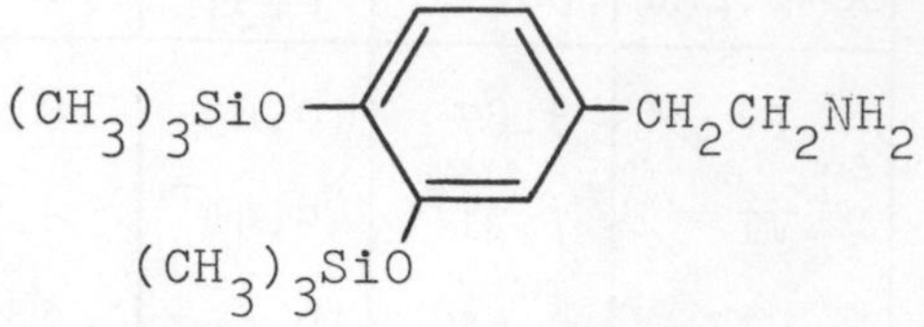

(XII)

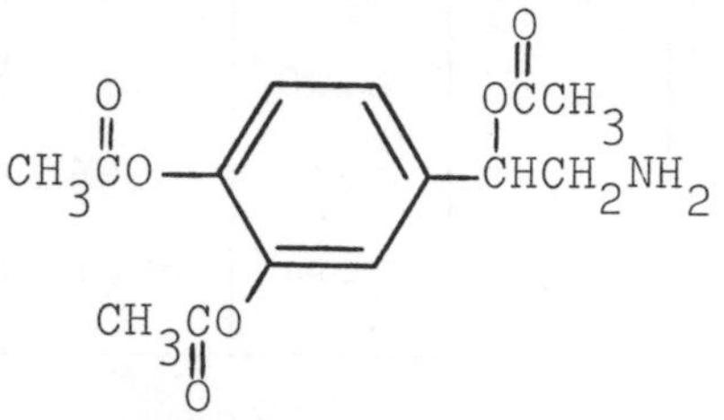

(XIII)

of Creveling et al. (69,70) who had shown that 3,4,
β-triacetyl (XIII), and 3,4,β-tri(trimethylsilyl)
(XIV) derivatives of norepinephrine caused prolonged
release of the parent catecholamine in mice brains.
However, as pointed out by Creveling et al. (69,70)
even though both XIII and XIV readily entered the CNS,
the derivatives survived as noncatechol entities for
long periods in the brain. For example, when H^3
tagged XIII was given I.V. to mice approximately 20%
of total brain radioactivity could be attributed to
catechol species while the remaining 80% was noncatechol species. In the hearts of the same animals the
reverse was the case, i.e., the derivative appeared to
be quickly converted to catechol species. This tends
to suggest that enzymatic regeneration of the norepinephrine from XIII may not be facile in the CNS.
Borgman et al. (71) have recently synthesized a series
of O,O-diacetyl derivatives of various dopaminergic
catecholamines including dopamine. The inability of
XI to antagonize oxotremorine-induced tremor in mice
(71), reserpine-induced depression (71) or to cause
hypothermia (71) in mice suggests that Pinder's proposal that XI should penetrate the CNS may be erro-
neous.

      The use of I.V. dopamine in the treatment of
shock (72,73) suggests that dopamine pro-drugs such as
XI and other O,O-diacyl (71,74) and amino acid amides
derivatives of dopamine (75) might provide useful,

orally bioavailable forms of dopamine for the treatment of shock. In the treatment of shock, peripheral
and not CNS levels of dopamine are desired.

Other examples of attempted chemical modification
intended to promote CNS absorption of amines include
the studies of Verbiscar et al. (76) with amphetamine,
Bjurulf et al. (77) with chlorphentermine and Kupchan
et al. (78) with normeperidine. Each study attempted
carbamoylation of the amine in an effort to (a) increase the lipophilicity of the amine by preventing
the ionization reaction. Penetration into the CNS
from blood has been correlated to lipophilicity and
the concentration of undissociated molecules in the
blood (79-81): and/or (b) prevent the metabolic action
of monoamine oxidase in brain capillaries (82). The
results with amphetamine and normeperidine were marginal. The carbamates of amphetamine did appear to
provide a prolonged release effect. The results of
Bjurulf et al. (77) with N-carbethoxychlorphentermine
(XV) or Oberex® (Draco), a pro-drug of the anorectic
agent chlorphentermine, showed that the pro-drug had a
"relatively prolonged effect which makes one dose in
the morning apparently sufficient."

$$Cl-\underset{}{\bigcirc}-CH_2\underset{\underset{CH_3}{|}}{\overset{\overset{CH_3}{|}}{C}}-\underset{\underset{H}{|}}{N}-\overset{\overset{O}{||}}{C}OC_2H_5$$

(XV)

Water soluble vitamins. Many of the water soluble B vitamins such as thiamine (vitamin B_1, XVI),
riboflavin (vitamin B_2, XVII) and pyridoxine (vitamin
B_6, XVIII) are highly polar and actively absorbed
agents.

Thiamine, being a water soluble compound with a
quaternary nitrogen, is poorly absorbed into the CNS
(83) and poorly absorbed from the GI tract (84-87).
Thiamine passes through these barriers because both
in CNS and oral absorption, it is actively absorbed.
However, active absorption processes are saturable
and/or easily inhibited. Inhibition of the oral absorption of thiamine by chronic alcohol consumption
has been implicated in Wernicke's encephalopathy (88)
and inhibited CNS absorption of thiamine has been implicated in the Leigh's disease (89,90). Thomson

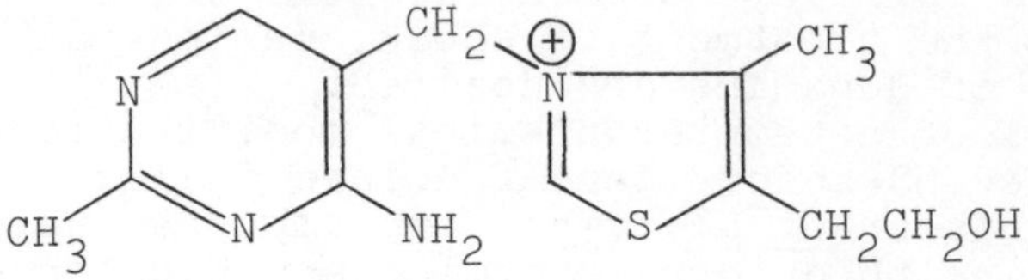

(XVI)

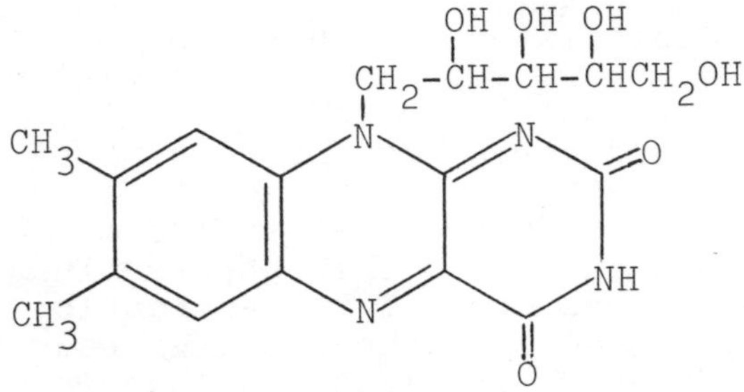

(XVII)

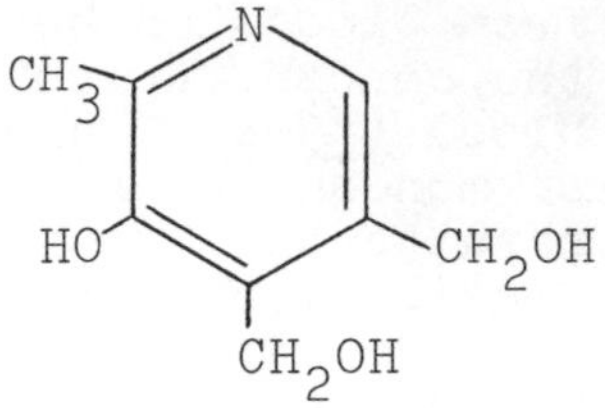

(XVIII)

et al. (88) have shown that chronic alcohol consumption and long dietary deficiency may reduce the intestinal absorption of thiamine. Thiamine undergoes
a rather unusual second ionization (Scheme V) to a
thiolate ion (XIX), involving the consumption of two
moles of hydroxide ion for each mole of thiamine.
Derivatization of XIX leads to many lipid soluble pro-
drugs of (a) the disulfide type, such as thiamine pro-
pyldisulfide (TPD, XX), thiamine tetrafurfuryldisul-
fide (TTFD, XXI) and O,O'-dibenzoylthiamine disulfide
(XXII); (b) diacyl type, such as O,S-diacetylthiamine
(DAT, XXIII); and (c) O,S- and S-carbonate esters of
thiamine, such as O,S-diethoxycarbonylthiamine (DECT,
XXIV). These and many other derivatives have been
synthesized in Japan since the early 1950's (91). The
synthesis of these derivatives was not necessarily
aimed at preferential GI or CNS absorption of thiamine
but was geared mainly to the possible use of these
lipid soluble thiamine derivatives as stable food additives. The polishing of rice had led to some thiamine deficiency in Japan. Thiamine itself could not
be used as a food additive for rice because it is too
water soluble, thus easily washed from rice. It is
also chemically unstable (92) and very poorly absorbed.

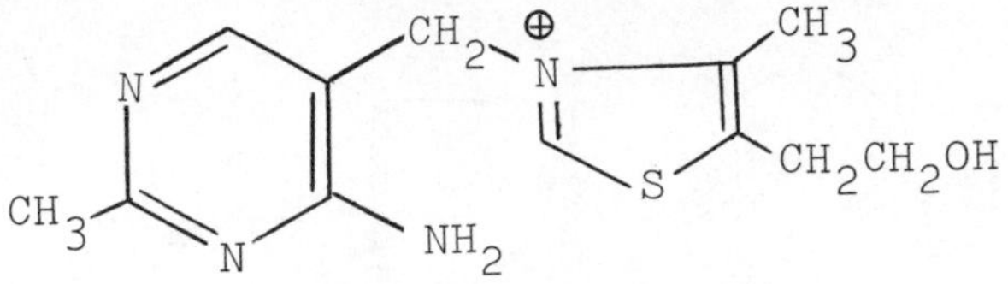

(XVI)

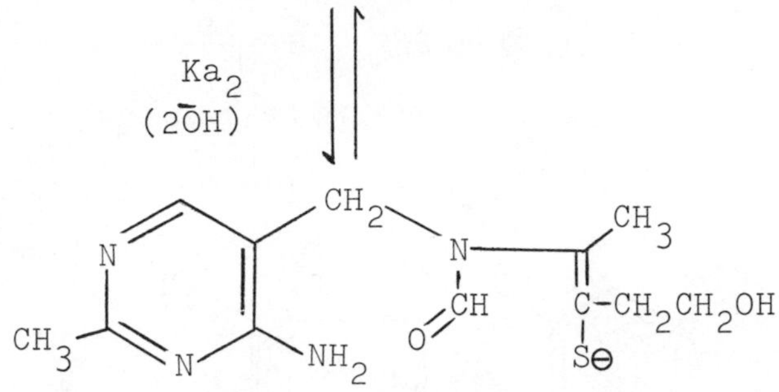

$$Ka_2$$
$$(2\bar{O}H)$$

(XIX)
Scheme V

Compounds like (XX-XXIV) and their homologues do not possess a quaternized nitrogen so allowing them to be passively absorbed from the GI tract. Each are quantitatively converted to thiamine once in the body (93). XXIII and XXIV and their homologues are converted to thiamine by thioesterases and esterases (93). The disulfide compounds (XX-XXII) and their homologues are converted to thiamine by a disulfide exchange mechanism implicating glutathione and glutathione reductase (94-97). Grode et al. (98) recently speculated that disulfide thiamine pro-drugs might be susceptible to interaction with serum proteins via a disulfide exchange reaction and precipitate antibody formation. Their results show that long term dosing of XXI in rabbits did not elicit antibody formation.

Thomson et al. (88) have presented some excellent data on thiamine blood and CNS levels in Wernicke's encephalopathy as well as lowered blood and CNS levels of thiamine in alcoholics having symptoms similar to but not necessarily suffering from Wernicke's disease. Their results show that XX on single oral dosing resulted in increased, and in some cases normal, red blood cell (RBC) transketolase activity in alcoholic, thiamine deficient patients while thiamine itself had

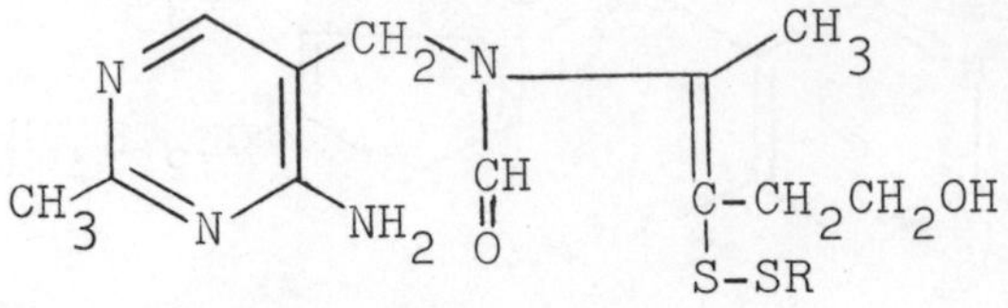

(XX): R = -C$_3$H$_7$

(XXI): R = -CH$_2$⟨furan⟩

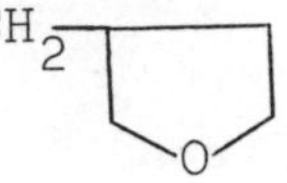

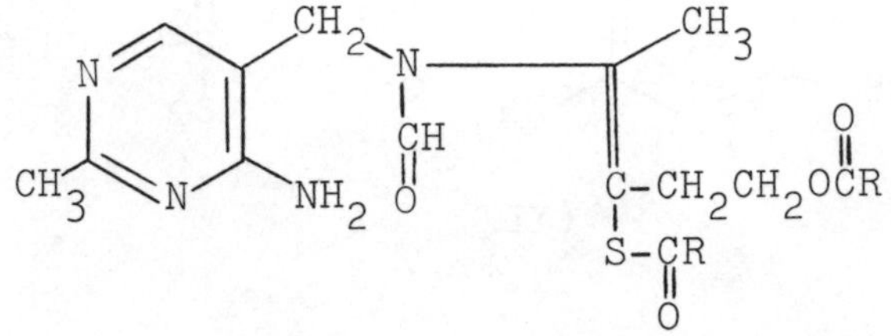

(XXIII): R = -CH$_3$

(XXIV): R = -OC$_2$H$_5$

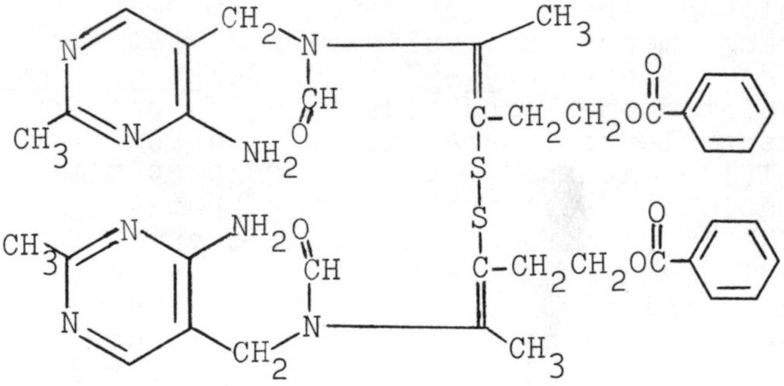

(XXII)

only a small effect on RBC transketolase activity.
Six hours after oral administration of XX, 5 of 6 alcoholic patients with Wernicke's disease and the accompanying bilateral rectus palsy showed complete re-

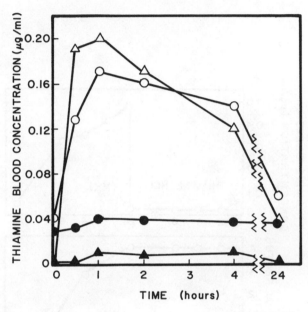

Annals of Internal Medicine

*Figure 2. Thiamine blood levels in malnourished alco-
holic patients with fatty livers (△) and in normal subjects
(○), given 50 mg of XX (open symbols) or 50 mg of thiamine hydrochloride (closed symbols) (88)*

mission of the occular palsy, with the sixth patient
showing an improved condition. Figure 2 gives the
thiamine blood level versus time profile for a 50 mg
dose of XX compared to an identical dose of thiamine

given to malnourished alcoholic patients with fatty
liver and normal subjects. Figure 3 is a comparison
of blood level and cerebrospinal fluid concentration
versus time profile and the accompanying clinical response for a group of thiamine deficient alcoholics
treated with thiamine for 25 hours and then treated
with an equivalent dose of XX.

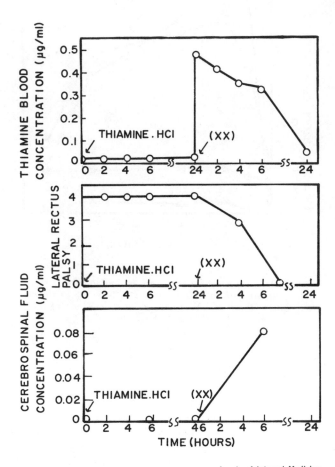

Figure 3.   Comparison of clinical and laboratory abnormali-
ties response to 50 mg of thiamine hydrochloride followed
by XX in thiamine deficient alcoholics (88)

Subacute necrotising encephalomyleopathy (SNE) or
Leigh's disease, a terminal disease afflicting children, has been suspected to be due to thiamine CNS
deficiency possibly caused by malabsorption of thiamine into the CNS. If thiamine CNS absorption is inhibited, the use of a passively absorbed lipid soluble thiamine pro-drug may prove useful. Pincus (89)
attempted to use XX in a number of Leigh's disease
cases with some degree of success. Temporary remis-
sions have been noted (89). Iwasaki (99) has studied

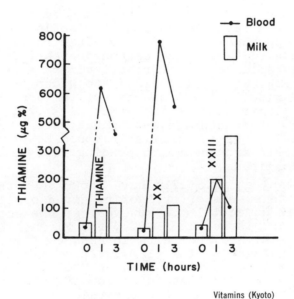

Vitamins (Kyoto)

*Figure 4.   Thiamine levels in milk and blood after
parenteral administration of 200 mg of modified thiamine compounds given S.C. to goats* (99)

the absorption of XXIII and XX into a lipid depot
(goat milk) after subcutaneous (S.C.) injection of
these derivatives to goats. Iwasaki's results are
shown in Figure 4. On the basis of this experiment,

XXIII would be expected to produce higher CNS levels of thiamine than XX or thiamine itself, especially in the presence of an inhibited thiamine CNS uptake mechanism. A preliminary clinical investigation using XXIII, at Loyola Medical Center, Maywood, Illinois, on a possible Leigh's disease case produced encouraging results (100).

For a complete review of thiamine pro-drugs, the paper of Kawasaki (93) should be consulted. For a summary of various synthetic procedures for preparing various thiamine pro-drugs, the reader is directed to the paper by Matsukawa et al. (91). The improved oral bioavailability of thiamine through dosing with various thiamine pro-drugs is well documented in the Japanese literature (91,93,99,102-113).

Chronic alcohol ingestion has also been shown to inhibit the active absorption of riboflavin, other actively absorbed water soluble vitamins (114,115), amino acids (116-118) and carbohydrates (116).

Fatty acid esters of riboflavin have been synthesized by Yagi et al. (119,120) "to widen the application of riboflavin to pharmaceutical and nutritional fields." Their results show that 2',3',4',5'-tetrapalmitate, -tetracaprate, -tetrabutyrate and -tetrapropionate esters of riboflavin could be hydrolyzed to riboflavin and the corresponding fatty acid by pancreatic lipase.

Shintani et al. (121) have shown that the di- and tripalmitate esters of pyridoxine given orally to mice had vitamin B_6 activity. However, if the esters were given intraperitoneally (I.P.), the vitamin B_6 activity was diminished. Results in rats confirmed the earlier findings in mice (122). It seemed that the palmitate esters required cleavage to pyridoxine before absorption and that injection of the esters resulted in their incomplete conversion to the pyridoxine. The triaminobenzoate ester of pyridoxine has also been prepared (123) as a possible pro-drug form of pyridoxine.

Lipophilic derivatives of ascorbic acid, such as 6-palmitoylascorbic acid (124,125) and 6-stearoylascorbic acid (126,127), have been synthesized as lipophilic antioxidants for nonaqueous formulations. Various mono- and polyacyl derivatives of ascorbic

acid have been synthesized with the view to increase
the aqueous stability of ascorbic acid. The weak
vitamin C activity of the 2,3,5,6-tetracetyl derivative administered orally has been noted (128) while
6-benzoyl (129-132), 6-stearoyl (126,127), 6-lauryl
(126,127) and some diacetyl derivatives have vitamin
C activity equivalent, but not superior, to ascorbic
acid. However, as will be discussed later, the 2-
and/or 3-acyl derivatives are more chemically stable
than ascorbic acid itself. The lipophilic 6-palmi-
toyl derivative is used as a lipophilic antioxidant.

   Nucleosides and nucleotides. Another group of
highly polar, poorly lipophilic molecules with resulting poor permeability characteristics are structural
analogs of the natural purine and pyrimidine nucleosides (133). These compounds can interfere with nucleic acid synthesis and the synthesis of proteins
and carbohydrates. The routine use of the nucleoside
analog, 6-azauridine (XXV), in the treatment of neoplastic diseases and psoriasis was impractical because of its poor oral bioavailability. The poor
bioavailability can be attributed to the poor permeability characteristics of XXV and/or metabolism of

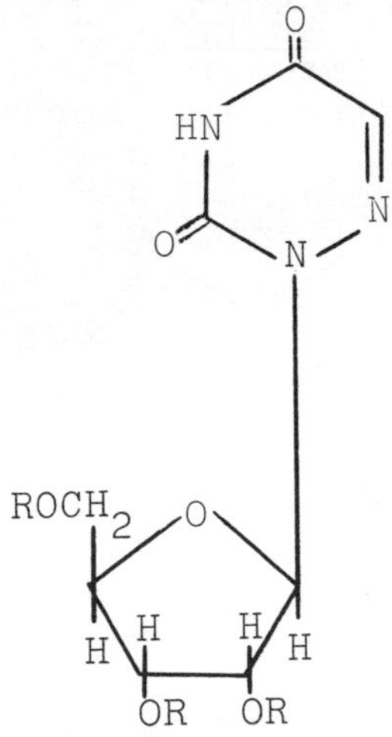

(XXV):   R = -H
(XXVI): R = $-COCH_3$
(XXVII): R = $-COC_6H_5$

XXV during the absorption process. The synthesis of
various esters of XXV such as 2',3',5'-triacetyl-
(XXVI), and 2',3',5'-tribenzoyl-6-azauridine (XXVII) as
well as other mono- and polyacyl derivatives was carried out in an effort to obtain an orally bioavailable
form of XXV (134-139). XXVI on injection in patients
suffering from various neoplastic diseases (140) was
found to be excreted in the urine as 6-azauridine (29-
77%) and monoacetyl-6-azauridine (4-19%). The treatment of psoriasis with oral doses of XXVI of 250
mg/Kg/day proved successful (141). XXVI given orally
to rats showed antifertility properties similar to XXV
with the added advantage that XXVI was orally absorbed
(142).

Welch (134) has stated that XXVI can be given
orally every 8 hours and is completely absorbed. On
oral dosing, XXVI is excreted 80% as XXV and 17% as its
5'-acetyl derivative with only traces of XXVI excreted.
Orally administered XXVI caused the same clinical effects as a molar equivalent dose of XXV given I.V.

The poor oral bioavailability of the nucleoside,
psicofuranine, (XXVIII), has been attributed to the
basicity of its 6-amino group, and its nonlipophilic
character (143). Various acetate esters of XXVIII were
prepared including the tetraacetate ester (XXIX). Oral
CD_{50} studies with S. hemolyticus infected mice showed
XXIX to be twice as effective as the parent compound
XXVIII. Figure 5 gives human serum levels of XXVIII as

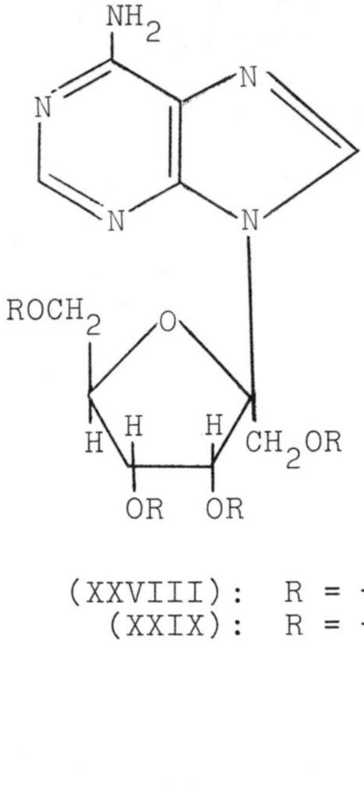

(XXVIII): R = —H
(XXIX): R = —COCH$_3$

a function of time after oral dosing with XXVIII and
XXIX. The poor bioavailability of XXVIII from an oral
dose of XXVIII was confirmed and the superiority of
XXIX as an orally available form of XXVIII demonstrated. Hoeksema et al. (143) state that the higher solubility of XXIX relative to XXVIII in chloroform (>150

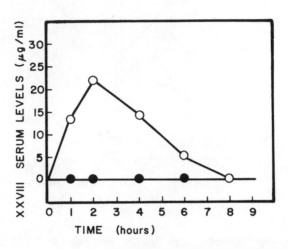

*Figure 5.   Serum levels in humans of XXVIII as a
function of time after 1.5 g oral dosing of XXVIII
(●) or XXIX (○) (143)*

mg/ml compared to 0.007 mg/ml), while maintaining a
reasonable aqueous solubility (3 mg/ml compared to
13 mg/ml), strongly suggested that the superior oral
availability of XXVIII from XXIX can be attributed to
the increased lipophilic character of XXIX.
     Cyclic 3',5'-adenosine monophosphate (XXX), a po-
lar nucleotide regulator of glycogenolysis, has been
acylated by Posternak et al. (144). The dibutanoyl
derivative, N^6-2'-O-dibutanoyladenosine-3',5'-mono-
phosphate (XXXI), given I.V. to dogs showed a greater
hyperglycemic activity than XXX itself. Two other derivatives, the N^6-butanoyl (XXXII) and the N^6-octanoyl
(XXXIII) derivatives, also showed superior and pro-

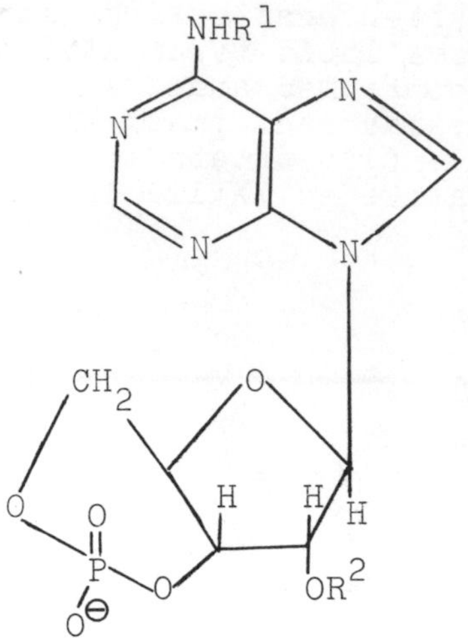

$$(XXX): \quad R^1 = R^2 = -H$$
$$(XXXI): \quad R^1 = R^2 = -COC_3H_7$$
$$(XXXII): \quad R^1 = -COC_3H_7, \quad R^2 = -H$$
$$(XXXIII): \quad R^1 = -COC_7H_{15}, \quad R^2 = -H$$

longed hyperglycemic activity compared to XXX. Posternak et al. (144) attributed this greater activity
to increased entrance into cells and/or the resistance
of the derivatives to inactivation by phosphodiester-
ases.

The acetate, formate and propionate esters of 9-
(β-D-arabinofuranosyl)adenine have been synthesized as
orally available forms of the parent drug (145). Ada-
mantoyl esters of various deoxyribonucleosides (specifically the 5' esters) have been prepared by Gerzon et
al. (146). Although the authors attribute the activity of the 5'-adamantoyl esters to the intact ester,
the possibility that the esters were acting as pro-
drugs of the parent nucleoside was not excluded.

Other polar compounds. The large difference between effective oral and I.V. doses of many quaternary
ammonium drugs has been attributed to the incomplete
oral absorption of quaternary compounds (147,148).
The oral absorption of quaternary ammonium compounds
from the GI tract has always presented a problem. At
least one quaternary compound, thiamine, has been
shown to be actively absorbed (84).

Levine <u>et al</u>. (<u>149</u>) were able to show that intra-molecular cyclizations could be used to overcome this problem. Table II shows four compounds. Compound XXXV under physiological conditions found in the plasma and intestinal tract is converted to XXXIV, the quaternary compound, via an intramolecular nucleophilic reaction. Similarly, XXXVII is converted to XXXVI. The absorption figures quoted in Table II were from <u>in situ</u> intestinal loop experiments and do not reflect the concentration of quaternary compounds actually appearing in the blood stream. As can be seen

TABLE II

Compound	% Absorbed After 3 Hours
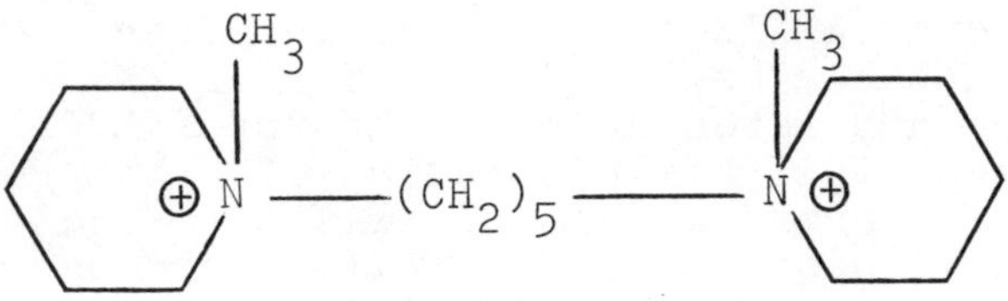 (XXXIV)	14
$Br-(CH_2)_5-\overset{\overset{\displaystyle CH_3}{\displaystyle |}}{N}-(CH_2)_5-\overset{\overset{\displaystyle CH_3}{\displaystyle |}}{N}-(CH_2)_5-Br$ (XXXV)	56
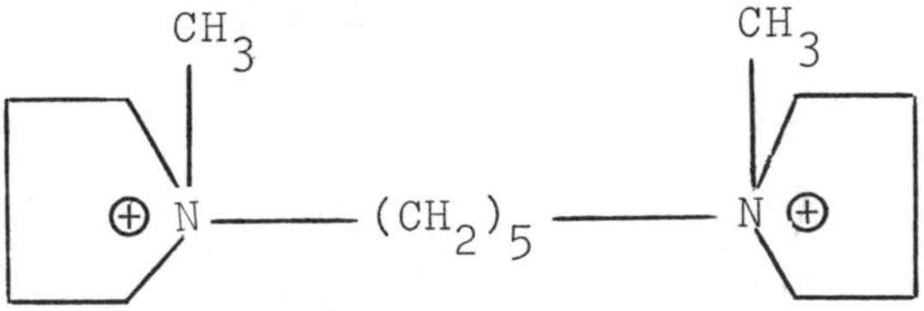 (XXVI)	16.8
$Cl-(CH_2)_4-\overset{\overset{\displaystyle CH_3}{\displaystyle |}}{N}-(CH_2)_5-\overset{\overset{\displaystyle CH_3}{\displaystyle |}}{N}-(CH_2)_4-Cl$ (XXXVII)	21

seen from the Table II, the quaternary compounds were
poorly absorbed because of their low lipid solubility
while the tertiary amine derivatives were better absorbed.   Studies (149) of the urinary elimination products after dosing with the tertiary amine precursors
showed that metabolic pathways other than conversion
to the quaternary compounds were occurring. As a result, the superior absorption characteristics of the
tertiary amine precursors did not necessarily reflect
increased blood levels of quaternary compounds.
     The mechanisms describing the intramolecular cy-
clizations of ω-haloalkylamines to their quaternary
analogues have been discussed by Streitwieser (150)
and Kusnetsov et al. (151). While Levine et al. pio-
neered the possible use of intramolecular cyclization
of the ω-haloalkylamines to their quaternary analogues,
Ross and coworkers (152-157), in a series of studies,
have attempted to utilize this concept more fully.
Ross and Fröden (152) studied the absorption and formation of XXXVIII from XXXIX in mouse brain after I.P.
administration of XXXIX. The I.P. injection of XXXVIII
itself did not give any detectable amounts of XXXVIII
in the brain, whereas I.P. administration of XXXIX resulted in substantial brain levels of XXXVIII.   The
quantitative conversion of XXXIX to XXXVIII in mouse
brain homogenates was also observed.   The purpose of
the study was to effect CNS absorption of a quaternary

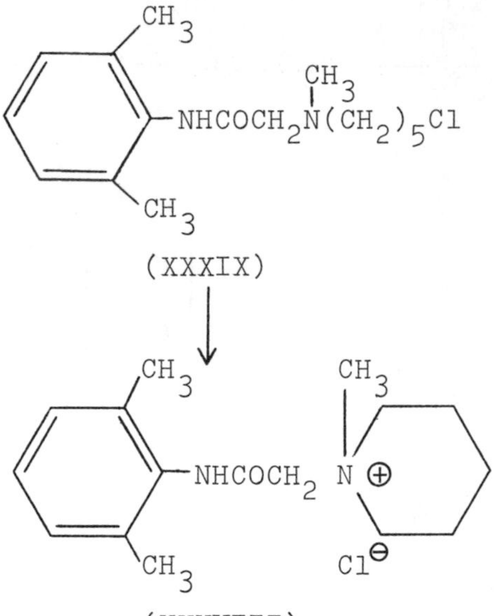

(XXXIX)

(XXXVIII)

compound by the administration of its tertiary ω-halo-
alkylamine precursor. The study of the elimination of
quaternary compounds from the CNS has been limited by
absorption, i.e., the study of elimination is difficult if it has never been established that the quaternary compound was effectively absorbed in the first
place. The very long elimination half-life of XXXVIII
from the brains of mice, approximately 30 hours, demonstrates the poor elimination of in situ formed polar
materials from the CNS. These results are consistent
with the findings of a long elimination halflife for
the polar and charged in situ formed acetate anion
elimination from the CNS (545).

Ross and coworkers (155) have subsequently studied the various parameters affecting the cyclization
of ω-haloalkylamines to their quaternary derivatives.

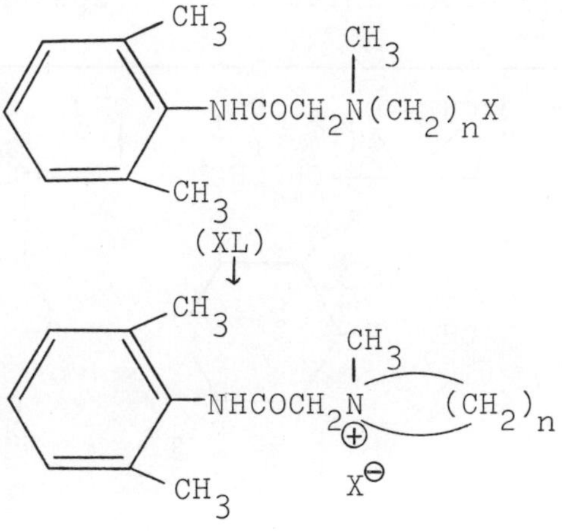

(XL)

↓

(XLI)

Scheme VI

Scheme VI was the general reaction studied. The duration and intensity of local anesthesia using in vivo
and in vitro tests, for both XL and XLI, were studied.
Chemical studies of the effect of n and -x on the conversion of XL to XLI and the local anesthetic activity
of both the tertiary analog itself and the formed quaternary compound suggested that the formed quaternary
compounds contribute to the duration of the anesthesia
(155,157). The local anesthetic effects of XL and XLI
on the sciatic nerve of guinea pigs, in vivo, and
frog, in vitro, showed that sustained local anesthetic
activity occurred for compounds where n = 5 and x =

-Cl or -Br. Apparently the prolonged activity was
well correlated with the extremely slow elimination of
the in situ formed quaternary compound from the sciatic nerve (157) and the concentration of the quaternary
compound in the nerve. Similar studies with bretylium
related derivatives (153), xylocholine related derivatives (154) and troxonium related derivatives (156)
have also recently been published.

The poor oral bioavailability of many antibiotics,
such as ampicillin (158-164), erythromycin (165-167),
oleandomycin (168) and lincomycin (169,170) has been
attributed to both their polar character as well as
metabolism in the GI tract, GI mucosa or liver during
absorption. The poor bioavailability of ampicillin as
compared to a number of pro-drug forms of ampicillin
will be discussed by Dr. Sinkula.

The antibiotic, oleandomycin (XLII) was found to
have a fairly broad anitbacterial spectrum and to be

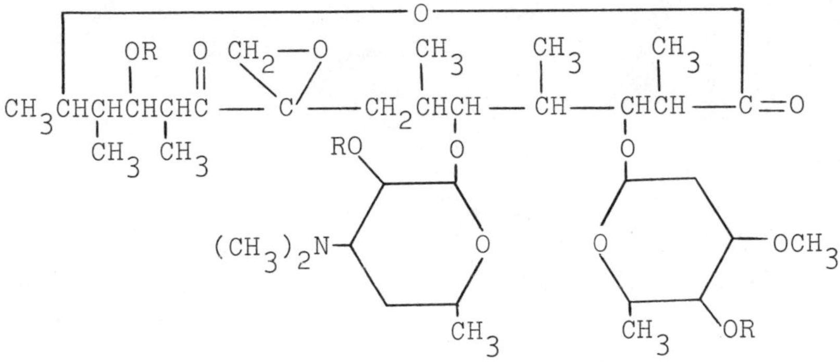

(XLII):   R = -H
(XLIII): R = -COCH₃

effective both orally and parenterally (171). It was
subsequently shown that its triacetyl derivative, tri-
acetyloleandomycin (XLIII) was more effective orally
than the parent compound (168,172-175). This increased effectiveness was attributed to the greater
bioavailability of XLII from XLIII than from XLII itself (See Figure 6). Clemer et al. have shown that
XLIII has some antibacterial activity of its own
against S. aureus and S. lutea but that the activity
was only 25% that of oleandomycin free base (172).
After ingestion of XLIII, XLII is detected in urine

along with 3-acetyloleandomycin, (major metabolite),
1-acetyloleandomycin and 1,3-diacetyloleandomycin (intermediate metabolites) and 2,3-diacetyloleandomycin
(minor metabolites).

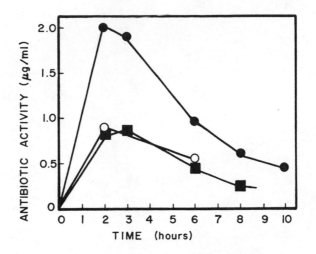

Antibiotics Annual

Figure 6.   Antibiotic activity vs. *time curve in human
beings given 500 mg XLII* (○), *500 mg XLIII* (●), *and
250 mg XLIII* (■). *Activity expressed in terms of XLII
base* (168).

The oral bioavailability problems of erythromycin
(XLIV) are well established (165-167). Esterification
of XLIV at the 2' position, (i.e., R_2 = -COR_3 where
R_3 = alkyl, aryl, alkoxy or -$(CH_2)_nCOOR_4$ where R_4 =
alkyl group) to give various esters was done with the
expressed purpose of lowering the aqueous solubility
of the erythromycin in an attempt to decrease its
bitter taste. Many of these esters on oral dosing
gave superior or equivalent blood levels to erythromycin base (176-181). The propionate ester in particular was considered to give superior levels of erythromycin when compared to erythromycin. There is
some discussion as to whether the conversion of the
2'-propionate ester to erythromycin is complete in

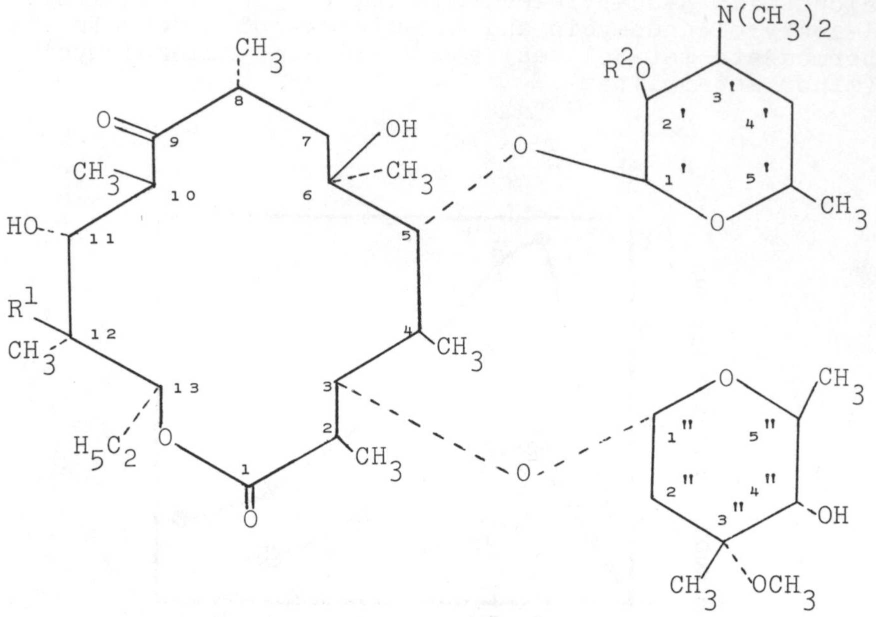

(XLIV):   erythromycin A, R^1 = -OH,
                                R^2 = -H
          erythromycin B, R^1 = -H,
                                R^2 = -H

vivo. Esterification of erythromycin at the 2', 4",
and 11 positions resulted in significant increases in
the lipophilicity of the molecules. Whether these
esters revert to the parent compound, maintain activity of their own, or impart any real advantage over
erythromycin itself is a currently controversial topic
(180,182). The ability of a number of erythromycin
esters and salts to mask the bitter taste of erythromycin will be discussed later.

     The polar antibiotic, lincomycin (XLV) has been
esterified at the 2 and 7 position (XLVI) in an
attempt to produce a tasteless form of XLV suitable
for pediatric dosing (183-185). Obviously the biological properties of XLVI, such as absorption characteristics and regeneration of the parent compound,
also need to be optimized. Good activity for 2-acyl
and 2-alkoxycarbonyl derivatives were noted in S.
aureus infected mice. The maximum activity was noted
for C_4 through C_{16} esters with median chain length
esters having the better activity (184). The

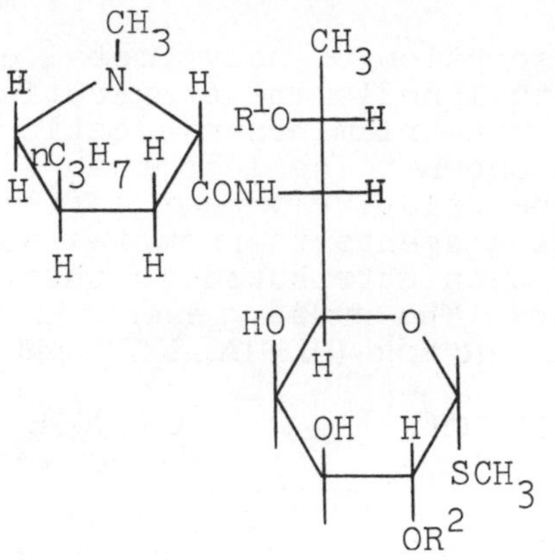

(XLV): $R^1 = R^2 = -H$

(XLVI): R^1 and/or R^2 = acyl or
alkoxycarbonyl substituent

2,7-dicarbonate esters were found to be inactive in
vitro but had in vivo activity after S.C. injection and
oral dosing in S. aureus infected mice. A number of
the derivatives (both acyl and carbonate esters) were
shown to achieve the original objective of the authors,
i.e., a tasteless lincomycin derivative with in vivo
activity comparable to lincomycin base (185).

Málek et al. (186) have attempted to increase delivery of polar antibiotics such as penicillin to pulmonary tissue and lymph nodes by derivative formation.
The authors argue that delivery to the lymphatic system might be achieved if drugs such as streptomycin,
neomycin and viomycin were associated as macromolecular
salts with carboxyl, sulfonyl or phosphoryl high molecular weight polymers. They conclude that these macro-
molecules, with their colloidal properties, have a high
affinity for the lymphatic system. The authors prepared a number of macromolecular salts of the various
antibiotics (the authors termed the resultant salts
"antibiolymphins") including (a) polyacrylate salts,
(b) salts with sulfonyl and phosphorylated polysaccha-
rides, and (c) salts with natural polycarboxylic acids
of the polyuronic and polysaccharide series. After
I.M., I.P., I.V., and intraplural administration of the
macromolecular salts of streptomycin, neomycin and viomycin, levels of the various drugs in the lymphatic
system appeared to be higher than levels obtained from
administration of an equivalent dose of the nonderiva-

tized drug.

The oral absorption of heavy metal chelating agents such as ethylenediaminetetraacetic acid (EDTA, XLVII) and diethylenetriaminepentaacetic acid (DTPA, XLVIII) had been shown to be less than 4% of the total dosage (187). The relatively poor effectiveness of a number of chelating agents to promote radioactive metal mobilization has been attributed to their poor permeability characteristics. The chelating agents (2-hydroxyethylenediamine-N,N,N-triacetic acid (HEDTA, LXIX) and N,N'-bis(2-hy-

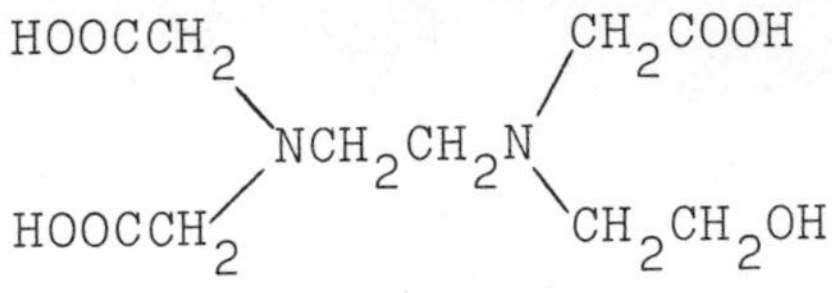

HOOCCH$_2$ ... CH$_2$COOH
NCH$_2$CH$_2$N
HOOCCH$_2$ ... CH$_2$CH$_2$OH

(XLIX)

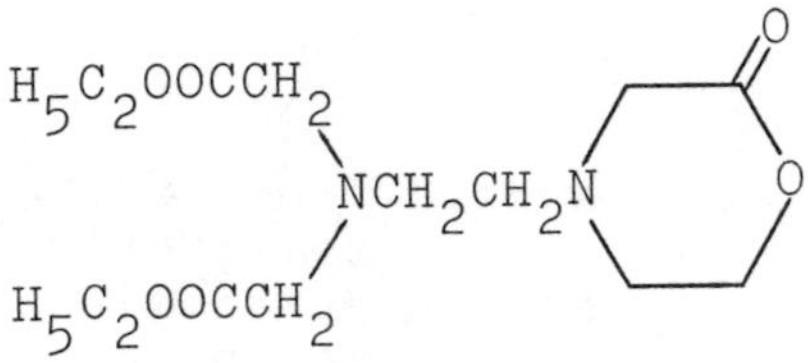

H$_5$C$_2$OOCCH$_2$
NCH$_2$CH$_2$N
H$_5$C$_2$OOCCH$_2$

(LI)

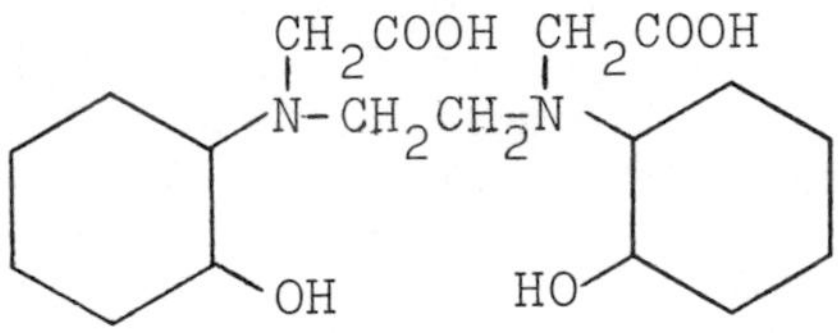

CH$_2$COOH   CH$_2$COOH
N–CH$_2$CH$_2$N
OH   HO

(L)

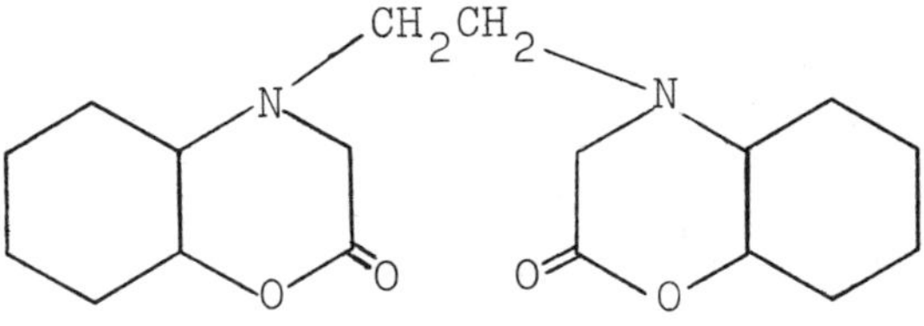

CH$_2$CH$_2$
N   N

(LII)

droxycyclohexyl)-ethylenediamine-N,N'-diacetic acid
(DOC, L) have been derivatized to the less polar compounds LI and LII respectively. After I.V. administration of LI, mobilization of various radiometals from
the liver of Ce^{144} dosed cats was far superior to an
equivalent dose of XLIX. LI administered orally was as
efficient at radiometal mobilization as an equivalent
I.V. dose of LI. The increased oral bioavailability
and increased permeability to various organs of LI and
LII were attributed to the less polar nature of the derivatives and their ready conversion to the parent compound . The increased mobilization of radiometals by
LI was attributed to the formed XLIX because LI was
shown to have no heavy ion chelating capacity (188).

   Opthalmic absorption of epinephrine. The highly
polar adrenergic agent, epinephrine (IX), is useful in
the treatment of glaucoma. As demonstrated earlier,
less than 1% of IX is present in its neutral form at
physiological pH. Acylation of the phenolic hydroxy
groups to give the dipivalyl derivative (LIII) was
found to increase the therapeutic effectiveness of IX
by a factor of approximately 100 (to be discussed further by Dr. McClure). Even though the fraction of

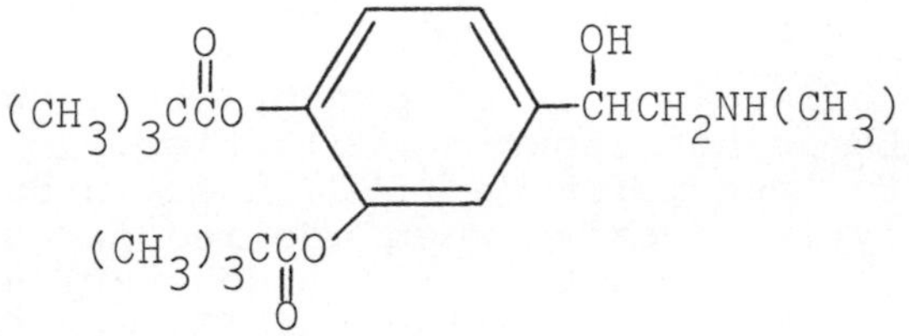

(LIII)

neutral molecule present at physiological pH should not
be greatly affected by the acylation, the lipid solubility of LIII is far superior to its parent compound,
IX. Since corneal absorption involves transport
through a lipoidal barrier, the greater lipophilicity
of LIII may account for its superior therapeutic effectiveness. The use of the dipivalyl ester was necessary
not only to increase the lipophilicity of the compound
but also to help guarantee adequate aqueous stability.

   Percutaneous absorption of polar drug entities.
The absorption of drugs into and through the skin is an
area of study which has achieved wide coverage but
which is not, as yet, fully understood. It is generally accepted that only neutral, relatively lipoidal drug

molecules can be absorbed percutaneously (194). The
work of Imai et al. (189) on the percutaneous absorption of the polar vitamin, ascorbic acid (LIV) and its
highly polar 3-phosphoryl ester (LV) tends to contra-
dict this generalization. The relevancy of this work

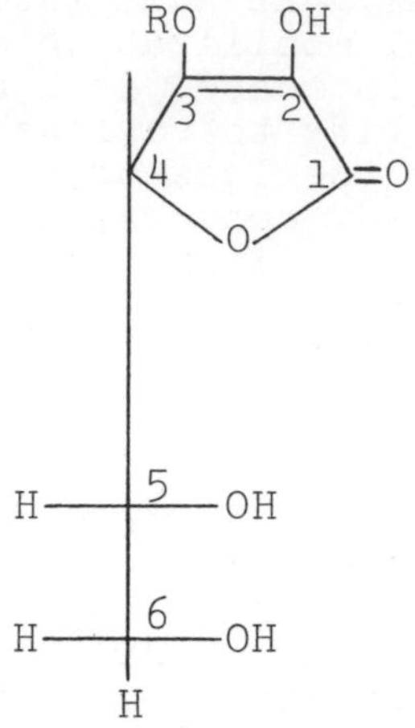

RO   OH

H————5———OH

H————6———OH

H

(LIV):   R = -H
(LV):   R = $-PO_3H_2$

and the true effectiveness of percutaneous absorption
of LIV from LV is not known at this time.
     The sulfa drug mafenide (LVI) used in burn therapy
was relatively ineffective when applied percutaneously
as its hydrochloride salt (LVII). However, application
of the acetate salt of mafenide (LVIII) was found to be
very effective in burn treatment (12-14). Mafenide is
marketed as Sulfamylon® (LVIII in a watermiscible
cream formulation) and Sulfamylon® hydrochloride solution (LVII as a 5% aqueous solution). The ineffective-
ness of the 5% aqueous solution of LVII in the treatment of burns has been discussed (190). The difference
in activity between LVII and LVIII is an interesting
problem. The pKa_1 of mafenide is 8.52 at 21°C (191).
A 5% aqueous solution of LVII would be expected to have
a pH of approximately 4.5. The pH of an aqueous film
of LVIII, regardless of concentration, would be expected to have a pH of approximately 6.6. Therefore, the
fraction of mafenide present in its neutral and presumably absorbable form, in a 5% solution of LVII is approximately 0.01% whereas the fraction present in an
aqueous solution of LVIII is approximately 1%. A model
for the absorption of mafenide into the skin is shown

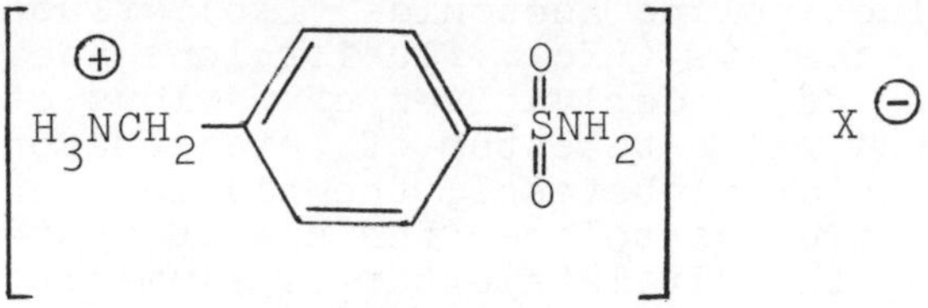

$$\left[\begin{array}{c} \overset{\oplus}{H_3NCH_2} - \underset{}{\bigcirc} - \overset{O}{\underset{O}{\overset{\parallel}{\underset{\parallel}{S}}}} NH_2 \end{array} \right] \quad X^{\ominus}$$

(LVII); $X^{\ominus} = Cl^{\ominus}$

(LVIII); $X^{\ominus} = CH_3COO^{\ominus}$

in Scheme VI. Whether LVI formation is favored will depend on whether $X^{\ominus}$ is a weak or strong base or whether LVII or LVIII is in buffered solutions. Since the acetate anion is a much stronger base than the chloride anion, the equilibrium is forced to the right favoring the formation of LVI. LVIII is considered a pro-drug of LVI, yet it is simply a salt of LVI and regeneration of LVI from LVIII involves simple dissociation.

Steroids are an area where the pro-drug approach has been apparently successfully utilized in attempts to promote topical or percutaneous absorption. Steroids such as triamcinolone (LIX), fluocinolone (LX) and fluclorolone have been derivatized to their acetonide derivatives (192), triamcinolone acetonide

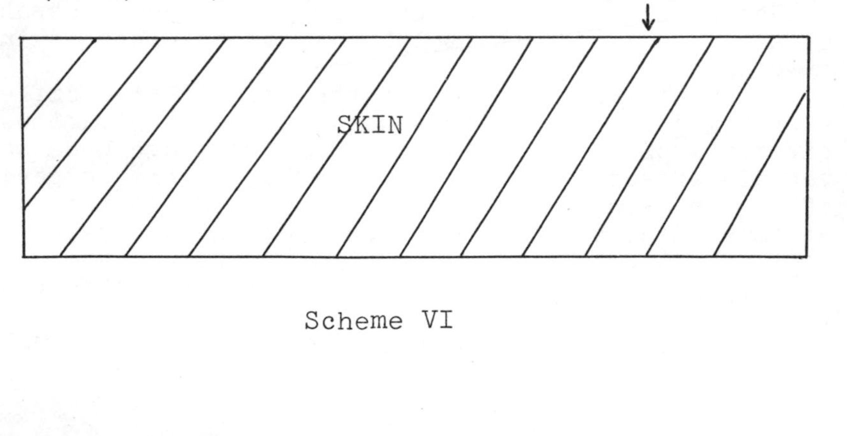

(LVII) or (LVIII)   (LVI)

Scheme VI

(LXa), fluocinolone acetonide (LXb), fluocinolone ace-
tonide-21-acetate (LXc), fluclorolone acetonide and
desonide. Ester derivatives of various other steroids
such as the valerate ester of betamethasone, the propionate ester of clobetasol, the pivalate and hexanoate
esters of flucocortolone, the acetate ester of hydrocortisone, the pivalate ester of flumethasone, the di-
propionate ester of beclomethasone, and the acetate
ester of methylprenisolene are examples of a few of
the corticosteroid esters in use (192,193).

Topical corticosteroids are used in the treatment
of inflammatory, allergic and pruritic skin conditions.
Whether any of the pro-drug derivatives exert any anti-
inflammatory activity of their own or whether they require conversion to the parent steroid for such activity can probably be argued.

Poulsen (194) has recently discussed formulation
factors affecting the percutaneous delivery of drugs.
As pointed out by Poulsen, there are many factors affecting the dermal delivery of a drug. It appears that
for solutions, gels, creams, etc., the diffusion of
drug across the skin barrier is rate limiting. In such
cases, the physical and chemical properties of the drug
to be delivered and the vehicle which contains the drug
are of paramount importance. In particular, the activity of the drug in the vehicle or the effective concentration of the drug in the vehicle determines, "the
driving force for diffusion from the vehicle" (194).

The diffusion coefficient, the activity of a drug
in a vehicle, and the partition coefficient of a drug
between the stratum corneum and the vehicle are all affected by the physical properties of a drug. Acetonide
formation of the dihydroxy groups in some steroids
(Scheme VII) or esterification of hydroxy groups in
other steroids generally results in an a priori increase in partition coefficient between the stratum
corneum and a hydrophilic vehicle. This causes an increase in the diffusion constant across human stratum
corneum and lowers the solubility of the steroid in the
hydrophilic vehicle.

Poulsen points out that the quantitative differences in anti-inflammatory activity between various derivatives of an agent is difficult to judge because of
vehicle effects (194). For example, in the comparison
of the anti-inflammatory activity of LXb to LXc (administered as a carboxypolymethylene gel containing
various ratios of propylene glycol/water as the solvent), LXb was found to be more active than LXc (human
vasoconstrictor assay) when the percentage of propylene
glycol in the gel was <55% but was found to be less

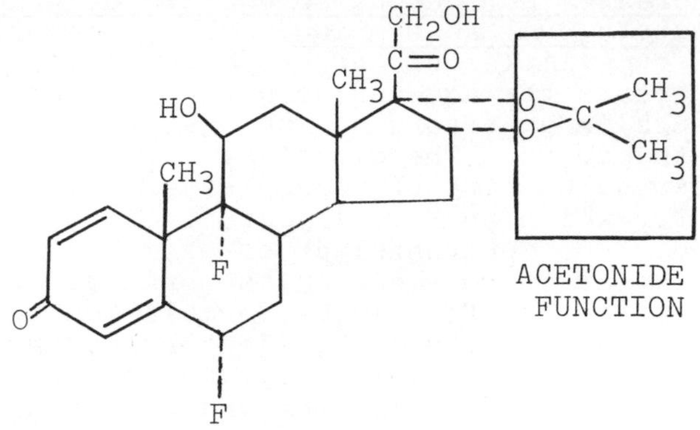

ACETONIDE
FUNCTION

(LXb)

Scheme VII

active when the percentage of propylene glycol in the
vehicle was >55%. These differences were attributed to
differences in solubilities of LXb and LXc in the vehicle as a function of propylene glycol concentration.
LXb (0.025%) was completely soluble in the vehicle when
the percentage of propylene glycol was >20-40% while
LXc (0.025%) did not dissolve completely in the vehicle
until the percentage of propylene glycol reached approximately 80%. The importance of vehicle composition, see Poulsen (194) for a complete discussion of
this problem, in the anti-inflammatory activity of steroids and their derivatives was recently re-emphasized
by the study of Barry and Woodford (192).

Maistrello et al. (195) have recently attempted to
quantitate the topical anti-inflammatory effects of
various steroidal agents administered as solutions in
2-(2-ethoxyethoxy)ethanol. The greater activity of LXa
relative to LIX was readily apparent.

The pro-drug approach has been successful in im-
proving the anti-inflammatory clinical efficacy of percutaneously administered steroids as can be seen by the
large number of steroids currently available as either
esters or acetonide derivatives (relative to nonderiva-
tized steroids). However, the role of the vehicle in
the success of these products has only recently begun
to be understood and fully appreciated (194).

To Increase the Aqueous Solubility of Drugs to
Help Facilitate Oral Absorption. Rather surprisingly,
there are few examples of the pro-drug approach being
used to increase the aqueous solubility of poorly water
soluble drugs in an effort to increase the oral absorp-
tivity of the drugs. The classical examples of improved water solubility of poorly water soluble drugs
are those for which an I.V. injectable form of the drug
was desired. The apparent lack of examples may be due
to the fact that improvement in the oral absorption of
a drug can often be effected by formulation techniques.
The oral bioavailability of 5,5-diphenylhydantoin,
nitrofurantoin, griseofulvin, digoxin, prednisolone,
etc., has been successfully improved by formulation
techniques.

The poor and erratic oral bioavailability of digoxin due to its low water solubility and formulation
variables has been well established (196-200). Higuchi
and Ikeda (201) have recently demonstrated that the
complex between hydroquinone and digoxin (2 digoxin:
3 hydroquinone) had a much higher dissolution rate than
digoxin itself.

Any crystalline material such as digoxin will have
a dissolution rate highly dependent on its aqueous
solubility as well as other variables defined in the
Noyes-Whitney equation (202). The energetics of the
dissolution process are determined by the breakdown of
intermolecular forces in the crystal lattice and the
solvent, both requiring energy, relative to the release
of solvation energy due to solute-solvent interactions.
The high melting point (265° with decomposition) of
digoxin strongly suggested that crystal lattice energy
played an important role in the poor aqueous solubility
of digoxin. The complexation of digoxin with a poly-
hydroxy compound such as hydroquinone might disrupt
this tight crystal lattice to form a complex with a
superior aqueous solubility. On dissolution, dissociation of the complex would rapidly release digoxin.
"Intrinsically more rapidly dissolving forms of digoxin
would provide greater assurance of more reproducible
and more bioavailable digoxin products" (201).

Use of digoxin derivatives such as its 4'''-methyl
derivative (203-205) and acylated derivatives such as
acetyldigoxin-α (206,207), acetyldigoxin-β (203,208-
211) have been promoted. The acylated derivatives of
gitoxin (212-214), as well as cyclic acetals and acetals of digitoxin, digoxin, and quabain have been of
interest (215). Although 4'''-acetyldigoxin (LXII) has
been shown to regenerate digoxin (LXI), 4''''methyldi-
goxin (LXIII) was not thought to revert to digoxin.

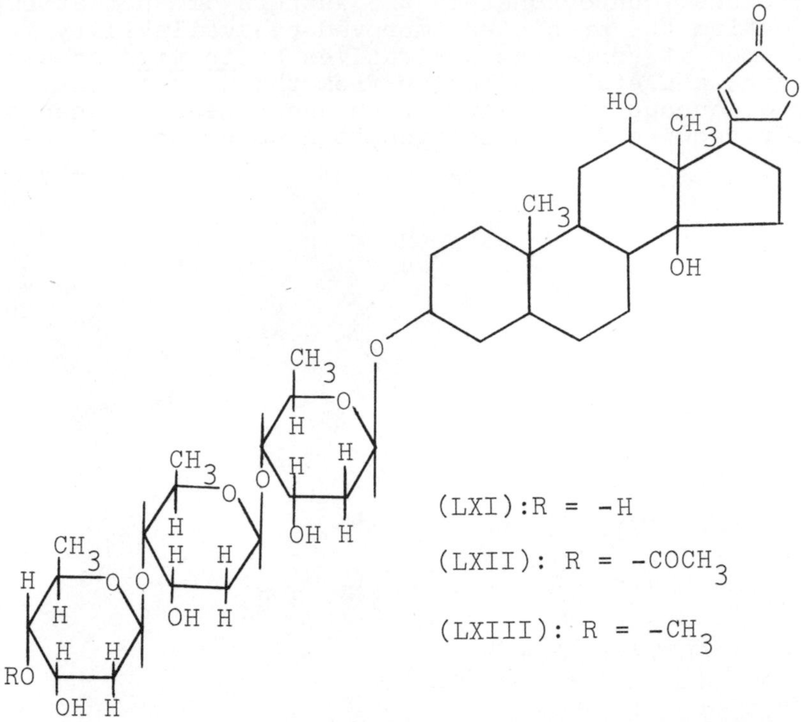

(LXI):R = -H

(LXII): R = -COCH$_3$

(LXIII): R = -CH$_3$

However, the studies of Rietbock et al. (204) confirm
that demethylation of LXIII does occur. Whether any of
these derivatives, monoalkyl (203-205) monoacyl (206-
214), or polyacyl (216), have any real advantage over
digoxin itself is debatable. White and Grisvold (217)
claim good oral absorption properties for LXII in cats
and LXII is marketed as Acylanid® (Sandoz) in the
United States.
     Recently, Hussain and Rytting (218) argued that
allopurinol (LXIV) owed its low water solubility of
0.78 mg/ml to strong intermolecular hydrogen bonding in
its crystal lattice. A melting point of 365° for LXIV
seemed to confirm this assumption. Disruption of the
crystal lattice by transient pro-drug formation was
suggested as a means of increasing the aqueous solubility of allopurinol. The authors synthesized 1-
ethoxyethyl-4-allopurinyl ether (LXV) and 2-tetrahy-
dropyranyl-4-allopurinyl ether (LXVI) and demonstrated
the improved dissolution rate from a constant surface
area pellet of LXV and LXVI when compared to LXIV.
LXV and LXVI were shown to regenerate LXIV under acidic

conditions. Unfortunately the authors did not attempt
to confirm the predicted improved bioavailability of
LXIV from its pro-drug derivatives by <u>in vivo</u> studies.
However, a useful conclusion from the work is that improved aqueous solubility of an agent need not necessarily require derivatization to a water soluble salt

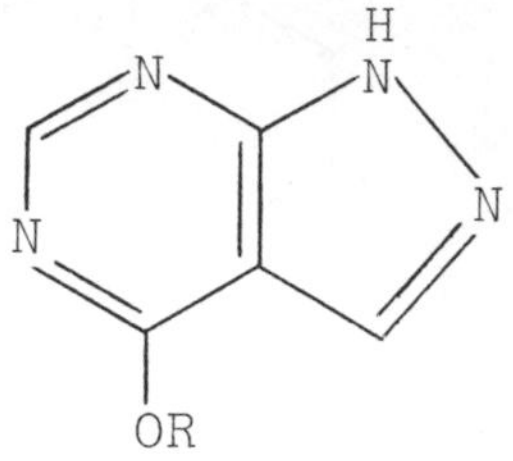

(LXIV):   R = -H

(LXV):   R = $-CH_2(CH_3)-OC_2H_5$

(LXVI):   R =

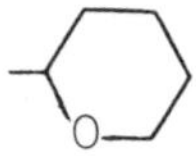

form of the drug. If the determining factor to poor
aqueous solubility is the strength of the crystal lattice of the drug, and this crystal energy is not sufficiently relieved by solvation energy on dissolution,
then disruption of the crystal lattice by pro-drug formation may provide a significant increase in aqueous as
well as lipid solubility.
     The strong crystal lattice energies of the hydan-
toins, 5,5-diphenylhydantoin and nitrofurantoin, and
various pro-drug forms of these drugs will be discussed
later by Stella <u>et al</u>.
     The antifungal agent, griseofulvin (LXVII), has
been shown to be poorly absorbed after oral administration to man as well as animals (<u>219</u>-<u>225</u>). The study by
Bates <u>et al</u>. (<u>226</u>) has shown that the absorption of
griseofulvin can be greatly enhanced by the concomital
administration of fats. It appears that the incomplete
bioavailability of LXVII is a function of its low water
solubility. This can be traced to its high lipophilicity, a contrast to the crystal lattice structure problems associated with the earlier examples. Fischer and
Riegelman (<u>227</u>) attempted to increase the aqueous solubility of LXVII by pro-drug formation. The derivatives

studied were griseofulvin-4'-alcohol (LXVIII), griseo-
fulvin-4'-oxime (LXIX), griseofulvin-4'-carboxymeth-
oxime (LXX) and griseofulvin-4'-hemisuccinate (LXXI).
In all discussions thus far, most of the derivatives
were esters of the parent compound where regeneration
of the parent compound was possible by the known presence and abundance of esterases in the body. The salt
and complex pro-drugs reverted to the parent compounds
by dissociation (a nonenzymatic process). In the case
of griseofulvin pro-drugs, the conversion of LXVIII to

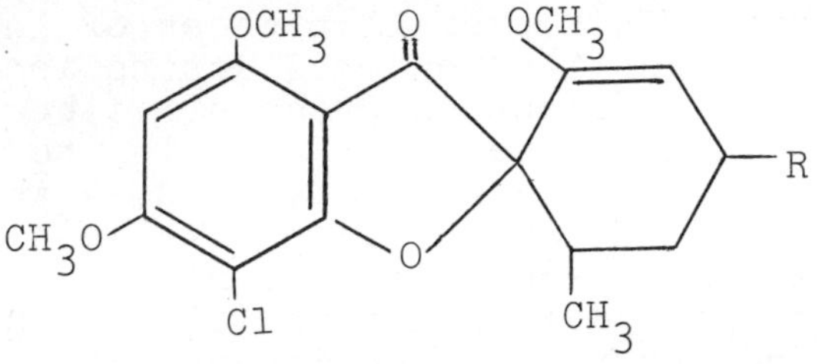

(LXVII):	R =	=O
(LXVIII):	R =	-OH
(LXIX):	R =	=NOH
(LXX):	R =	=NOCH$_2$COOH
(LXXI):	R =	-OCOCH$_2$CH$_2$COOH

LXVII requires an oxidative metabolism. On I.V. dosing
to a rabbit, the disappearance of LXVIII from the plasma of the rabbit had a half-life of 28 minutes whereas
the formed griseofulvin had a half-life of 70 minutes.
LXXI is converted to LXVII by esterase hydrolysis of
the ester function followed by oxidation of the formed
LXVIII. Oximes have also been shown to be enzymatically converted to the corresponding ketone (228).

     Although each of the LXVII pro-drugs had superior
aqueous solubilities when compared to LXVII (227),
none of the derivatives on oral dosing showed any superiority over LXVII itself. This was postulated to be
due to either incomplete conversion of the derivatives
to LXVII, concurrent metabolism to inactive metabolites, or elimination from the body before conversion
to LXVII was complete.

     To Help Stabilize Drugs Against Metabolism and/or
Hydrolysis During Oral Absorption. Many drugs are extremely active if administered parenterally but suffer
from the problem of incomplete absorption on oral

dosing. This incomplete absorption, as has already
been noted, can result from the drug being too polar or
poorly water soluble. A third possible reason for incomplete absorption is that the drug, if administered
orally, may be rapidly metabolized by enzymes secreted
into the GI tract, by bacteria in the GI tract, by enzymes encountered while passing through the GI mucosa,
and/or by the liver in its initial transit through the
liver before ever reaching the general circulation.
Examples of drugs poorly absorbed due to one or a combination of these processes have already been discussed, e.g., L-Dopa. This overall process of incomplete systematic availability on oral absorption due to
metabolism during the absorption process has been
termed the "first pass" effect (30-34). The term
"first pass" effect was originally defined as involving
only liver extraction (30). It has become less well
defined and is used generically to describe dose dependent bioavailability due to metabolism of orally administered drugs during the absorption process.
Magee et al. (229) have recently studied the in situ
absorption of various prostaglandins from the small intestine of rats. Although disappearance from the rat
lumen was fairly rapid for all the prostaglandins, very
little of the dose actually appeared in the blood
stream and only a small fraction of this "effectively"
absorbed dose was intact prostaglandin. The prostaglandin, 15-methyl $F_{2\alpha}$ (LXXII) and its methyl ester
(LXXIII) were studied. LXXII had an apparent absorption half-life of 60-70 minutes with approximately 2%
of the dose reaching general circulation but of that
only 0.8% was intact LXXII. When LXXIII was administered up to 7% of the dose reached general circulation, and 1.8% of the dose was present in serum as in-

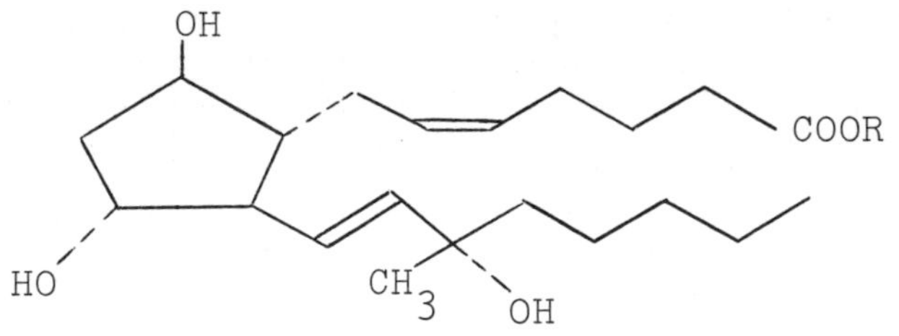

(LXXII): R = -H

(LXIII): R = -CH$_3$

tact LXXII with little or no detectable LXXIII. This
is a clear example of an agent, notoriously susceptible to metabolism, that was chemically modified to
partially overcome the "first pass" effect.

That esterification of prostaglandins inhibits
the metabolism of prostaglandins was clearly demonstrated by the greater activity of the methyl ester of
prostaglandin 15-methyl $E_{2\alpha}$ over the parent non-methyl
ester prostaglandin. The greater potency is attributed to a lengthening of the metabolic half-life (230)
of the ester form relative to the parent acid prostaglandin.

Another group of compounds which undergoes considerable metabolism during oral absorption are steroids.
The bioavailability of a number of steroidal drugs is
unknown because of analytical limitations of sensitivity and interference from natural steroidal hormones
in analyzing for absorbed intact steroid. Another
contribution to this unknown bioavailability is that
many of the steroids are probably metabolized to active agents.

Schedl et al. (231) showed that the rate of absorption of various steroids using the in situ rat intestinal loop experiment was rapid and inversely proportional to the number of hydroxy or polar groups
present in the molecule. This observation was confirmed when many of the steroids were acetylated and
the absorption rate of the acetylated versus the non-
acetylated steroids compared. Although many of the
steroids were found to be rapidly absorbed, the weak
oral potency of a number of the agents, e.g., testosterone, progesterone and desoxycorticosterone, which
were apparently well absorbed, the authors state that
the "pharmacologic activity of a steroid by the oral
route is independent of its absorption rate. Blood
levels of steroids following oral administration are
more a function of metabolic disposition than of absorption rate" (231). Acetylation may not only help
increase the absorption rate of these steroids but may
also provide a degree of metabolic protection.

Tanabe et al. (232) and Fried et al. (233) have
shown that 17α,21-acetonides of various corticosteroids have higher oral activity than their parent steroids on oral dosing. The study of Fried et al. (233)
demonstrated the higher activity of 16α,17α-acetonide
of triamcinolone (LXXIV) over the parent steroid
(LXXV). Gardi et al. (234) also observed that prednisolone acetonide (LXXVI) when administered orally and
prednisolone cyclopentylidenedioxy (LXXVII) when applied locally had greater activity than the parent

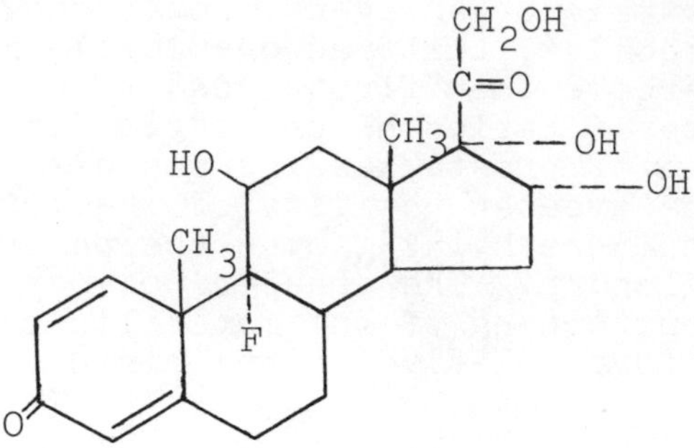

(LXXV)

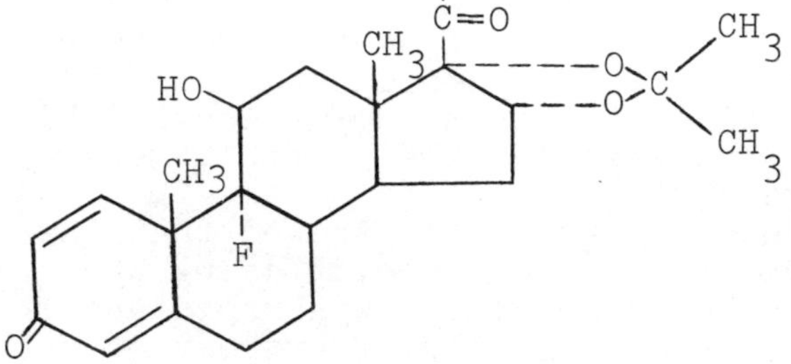

(LXXIV)

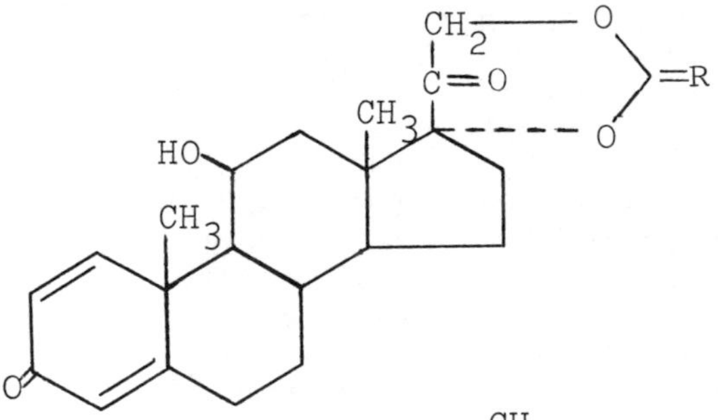

(LXXVI): R =

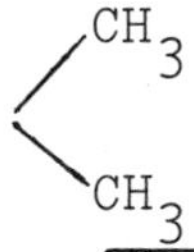

(LXXVII): R =

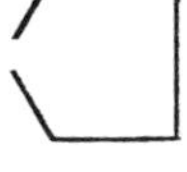

prednisolone. The antifertility, anti-inflammatory
compound 9α,11β,21-trichloro-16α,17α-(isopropylidene-
dioxy)-1,4,6-pregnatriene-3,20-dione, an acetonide derivative, was also shown to be orally active (235).

The steroid desoxycorticosterone (LXXVIII) is
very unstable and difficult to handle but its acetate
ester has been used parenterally in the treatment of
Addison's disease. LXXVIII as its acetate ester has
been found to be destroyed after oral administration
but when given sublingually was found to be useful in
the treatment of Addison's disease (236).

Gardi et al. (237) have recently demonstrated the
high oral activity of 1,3,5(10)-estratrien-17β-yl enol
ethers and acetals as new classes of orally and parenterally active estrogenic derivatives. The activity
is attributed to the in vivo regenerated estradiol.
Moreover the authors state that "the ether linkage
should be stable enough to survive the acidic gastric
medium and suitably delay the hepatic inactivation
after oral administration."

That catecholamines show poor absorption through
lipoidal membranes was established earlier in this
manuscript. "First pass" metabolism, primarily due to
conjugation (glucuronidation and/or sulfation), was
also mentioned as a primary means of limiting the systemic availability of catecholamines and other phenolic compounds. The narcotic antagonist naloxone
(LXXIX) has been shown to have low potency after oral
administration (238-241). The short duration of action of
LXXIX after parenteral dosing due to rapid metabolism
suggests that naloxone might be rapidly metabolized by
the liver and/or gastric mucosa on oral dosing, i.e.,
the poor oral activity results from a "first pass" effect. Linder and Fishman (240) synthesized a series
of sulfate and acetate esters of LXXIX and tested
their narcotic antagonist activity after oral and parenteral dosing in rats. The 3-acetyl derivative
(LXXX), 14-acetyl derivative (LXXXI) and 3,14-diacetyl
derivative (LXXXII) all showed good oral activity in
the morphine challenge test whereas LXXIX administered
orally was relatively ineffective. After I.V. administration, both LXXX and LXXXI were more potent than
LXXIX whereas LXXXII was slightly less potent than
LXXIX. These results suggest that the acetylation of
the 3 and/or 14 hydroxy groups of LXXIX blocked (or
partially blocked) the "first pass" metabolism of
LXXIX (probably sulfation and/or glucuronidation) by
protecting the hydroxy groups.

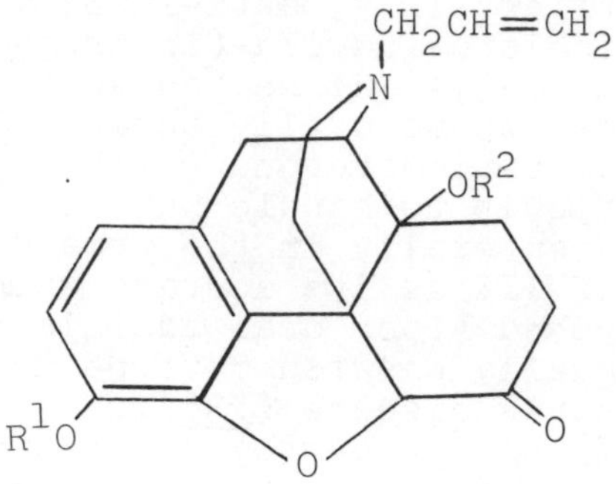

(LXXIX): $R^1 = R^2 = -H$
 (LXXX): $R^1 = -COCH_3$, $R^2 = -H$
(LXXXI): $R^1 = -H$, $R^2 = -COCH_3$
(LXXXII): $R^1 = R^2 = -COCH_3$

Way and Adler (242), in their review of morphine
(LXXXIII), morphine metabolites, and other narcotic
analgetics, state that the poor oral activity of morphine relative to its parenteral activity may be due
to the poor oral absorption of morphine. The essentially negative pharmacological activity of orally administered morphine in man can be interpreted as either
poor intrinsic absorption and/or "first pass" metabolism. Heroin or 3,6-diacetylmorphine (LXXXIV) exhibits

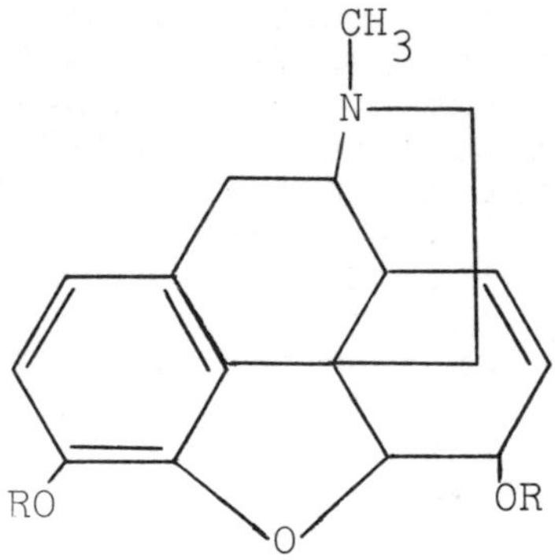

(LXXXIII): $R = -H$
(LXXXIV): $R = -COCH_3$

considerable if not somewhat irregular activity in man
after oral dosing which is again consistent with the
blocking (or partial blocking) of "first pass" metabolism. The rapid deacetylation of LXXXIV in all biological tissues, including the CNS, to LXXXIII and its mo-
noesters is well established (242). Kupchan et al.
(243) synthesized labile ether derivatives of morphine
and phenazocine and showed their activity to be less
than those of the parent compounds. Papers by Yoshimura et al. (244), Oguri et al. (245) and Mori et al.
(246) have confirmed the presence of glucuronide and
sulfate metabolites of morphine. Their results surprisingly show that the 6-glucuronide and 6-sulfate metabolites when injected S.C. in mice (246) give higher
potency and larger duration of analgetic activity compared to a comparable dose of morphine. As pointed out
by the authors, both the 6-glucuronide and 6-sulfate
are minor metabolites of morphine.

In a series of papers by Fields et al. (247-250),
various latentiated forms of thiols, amino-thiols and
2-acetamidoethanethiol were attempted to help reduce
the toxicity and/or improve activity, i.e., increase
availability, but with marginal success. Similarly,
Hartles et al. (251) and Siuda et al. (252) synthesized
and tested for activity a number of acyl and carbamate
derivatives of mafenide (LVI). Their objective was to
find orally active forms of LVI. LVI was shown to undergo rapid metabolism on oral absorption and it was
felt that N^4-acyl and N^4-alkoxycarbonyl derivatives
might prevent the rapid metabolism so resulting in adequate blood levels. Regeneration of LVI from its N^4-
acyl and N^4-alkoxycarbonyl derivatives was felt to be
too slow and inadequate to produce reasonable blood
levels of LVI.

Recently the tuberculostatic agent, p-aminosali-
cylic acid (LXXXV), has been shown to undergo "first
pass" metabolism due to N-acetylation (253). In efforts to obtain tasteless forms of LXXXV, various chemical and formulation modifications of LXXXV have been
attempted. Most of these modifications result in a
slower release form of LXXXV which is then more readily
and efficiently metabolized. However, an interesting
pro-drug of LXXXV, the calcium 4-benzamidosalicylate
(LXXXVI), which is quite water insoluble has been shown
to be as clinically effective on a molar basis as LXXXV
and yet tasteless (254,255). This appears paradoxial
in that most slow release forms of LXXXV provide incomplete bioavailability due to the "first pass" effect.
It appears that LXXXVI may provide a poorly soluble,
 tasteless form of LXXXV while circumventing "first

pass" acetylation (the aromatic group already being
acylated) and once in the body regenerates LXXXV. The
rate of deacylation of N-acyl derivatives of drugs
other than formyl derivatives and benzoyl derivatives
is poor. Chiou (256) has shown that deformylation of
4,4'-diformamidodiphenylsulfone (DFD, LXXXVII) to the
antimalarial agent, 4,4-diaminodiphenylsulfone (DDS,
LXXXVIII) by kynurenine formamidase of mammalian livers
does occur (see Scheme VIII).

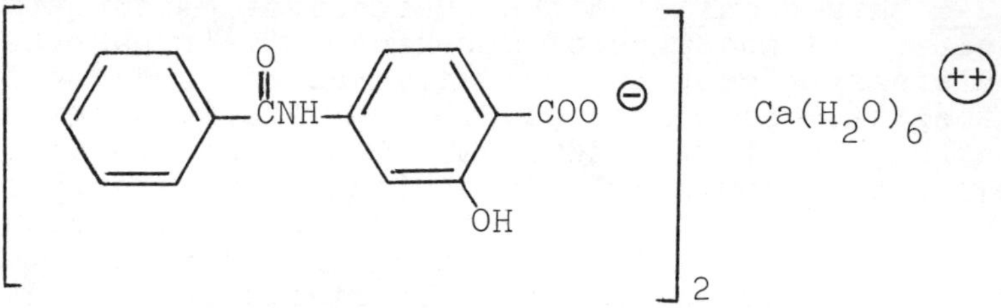

(LXXXVI)

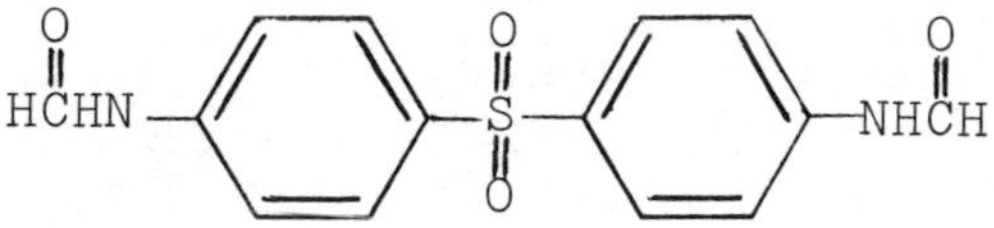

(LXXXVII)

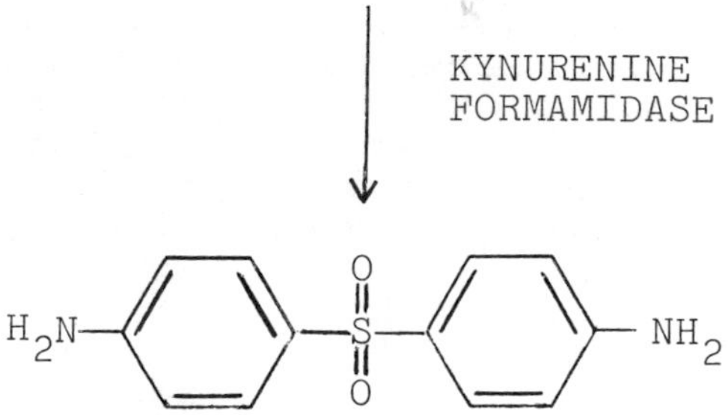

KYNURENINE
FORMAMIDASE

(LXXXVIII)

Scheme VIII

The Use of Pro-Drugs to Effect Sustained or Prolonged Release

Sustained release has usually been effected in pharmacy by the use of various dosage form changes such as coated slow release beads and granules, multiple layer tablets, and other formulation techniques (257). Many of the examples of pro-drugs causing sustained release incorporate a formulation technique combined with chemical modification ideas.

Stempel (257) has described the advantages of prolonged or sustained release products: (a) reduces the number and frequency of doses needed to be administered; (b) eliminates the "peak" and "valley" effects noted with conventional fast release preparations; (c) often reduces the total amount of drug needed to effect the desired pharmacological activity; (d) eliminates the problem of nighttime administration of drugs; (e) helps minimize the problem of patient noncompliance by decreasing the number of times a patient must remember to take their medication; (f) reduces the incidence of peak blood levels rising above the toxic blood levels; (g) reduces the incidence of GI side effects. To maintain an effective blood level of the very short half-lived drug cytosine arabinoside (LXXXIX), long term I.V. infusions of considerable inconvenience to the patient and nursing staff are needed. 5'-Acyl derivatives of LXXXIX (an immunosuppressive, antiviral and cytotoxic agent) as well as 2' and 3' esters have been synthesized and tested (258-262). When the slightly water soluble 5'-acyl derivatives (XC) were administered I.P. to mice as suspensions the pro-drugs dissolved slowly, gradually releasing XC to the circulation where the derivatives were enzymatically cleaved to LXXXIX allowing it to exert its pharmacological activity. Gray et al. (258) demonstrated a qualitative correlation between activity of the XC derivatives and decreasing aqueous solubility suggesting that the slow dissolution of the suspension of the 5'-esters was important. The slightly soluble esters such as the 5'-palmitate, 5'-stearate, 5'-benzoate and 5'-adamantoate were particularly impressive. The slightly water soluble but sterically hindered ester, 2,4,6-trimethylbenzoate and the sulfonate ester, 2,4,6-triisopropylbenzene sulfonate were less effective than the parent compound, presumably because of their slower enzymatic cleavage to the parent compound.

Probably the area in which the greatest effort has been made to effect sustained or prolonged release activity via the pro-drug approach has been in the area

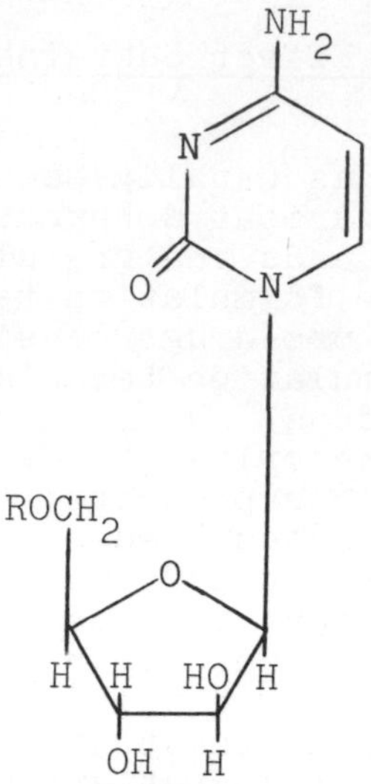

(LXXXIX):   R = -H
(XC):   R = acyl substituent

of steroid therapy. Recently Tanaka et al. (263) have
attempted to quantitate factors which affect the prolongation of activity of drug injected I.M. in oily
solutions. James et al. (264) showed that for a series
of testosterone (XCI) esters the biological halflife
for the release of testosterone and its esters from an
I.M. oil injection was closely related to the oil/water
distribution coefficient of the derivatives. The oil
used by James et al. (264) was ethyl oleate. It was
interesting to note that the homologous series of formyl through valeryl esters of testosterone had approximately equal solubility in the ethyl oleate showing
that the distribution coefficient was largely determined by the decrease in water solubility. Apart from
these interesting basic studies, the results of many
workers have shown that longer duration of action of
testosterone from an I.M. injection could be effected
by acylation of the 17β-hydroxy group (265-288). Increasing chain length of the acyl group effectively increased the duration of action, i.e., the testosterone
esters are thought to gradually leach out of the I.M.
injection site (oil based I.M. injection), regenerate
testosterone in the general circulation which then
exerts its androgenic activity (264).

Miescher et al. (265) were the first to promote the use of long chain esters of testosterone as depot forms of testosterone.   Ott et al. (276) have suggested that the β-cyclopentylpropionate ester of testosterone (XCII) injected I.M. in cottonseed oil was a superior ester form of testosterone when compared in a series of saturated and nonsaturated esters.   This conclusion was based on the relative growth of seminal vesicles in castrated rats after I.M. dosing of the various esters.   Similarly, Meier and Tschopp (284) using the growth of the capon crest as an indicator, showed that the undecylenate ester of testosterone (XCIII) was far superior in duration of action to the propionate, isobutyrate and n-valerate esters.   Voss (277) and Haack et al. (278) promoted the use of β-

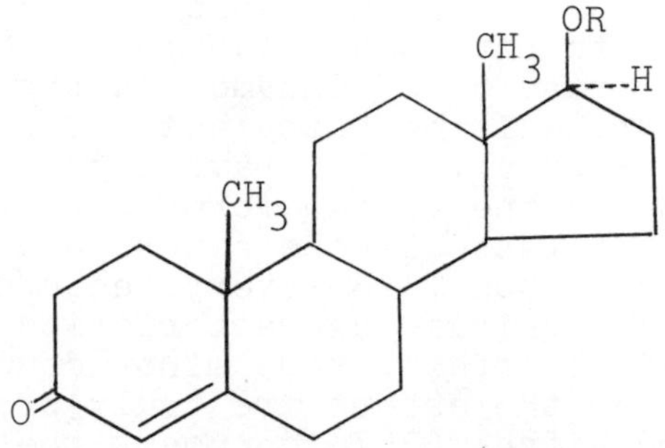

(XCI):   R = —H

(XCII):   R = —COCH$_2$CH$_2$⬠

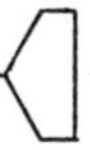

(XCIII):   R = —COC$_{10}$H$_{21}$

(XCIV):   R = —COCH$_2$COC$_9$H$_{19}$

(XCV):   R = —COCH$_2$CH$_2$-⬡

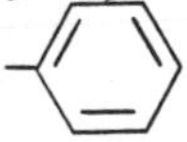

(XCVI):   R = —COC$_2$H$_5$

(XCVII):   R = —COCH$_2$CH$_2$-⬡-OC$_7$H$_{15}$

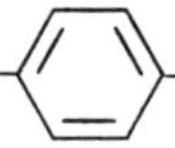

(XCVIII): R = —COC$_6$H$_{13}$

(XCIX):   R = —COC$_{15}$H$_{31}$

(C):   R = —COCH$_2$-⬡

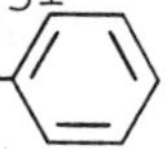

ketonic esters of testosterone, especially testosterone decanoylacetate (XCIV). Dekanski and Chapman (273)
felt that testosterone phenyl propionate (XCV) was as
effective as XCII but was far superior to the earlier
promoted testosterone propionate (XCVI). Diczfalusy
et al. (271) demonstrated the superiority of a series
of alkoxyhydrocinnamic acid esters of testosterone to
both XCV and XCVI. Para-heptyloxyhydrocinnamyltestos-
terone (XCVII), showing considerable activity over 90
days, appeared superior to XCV and XCVI.
     The study of Junkmann and Witzel (267) is the
most comprehensive review of depot forms of testosterone and other steroids. The enanthate (XCVIII), undecanoate (XCIII), and palmitate (XCIX) esters of testosterone all showed excellent prolonged activity.
     Evaluation of various other esters of testosterone
as depot forms of testosterone can be found (265-288).
It is interesting to note that Kishimoto (289) has recently noted the presence of enzymes in the CNS that
are capable of synthesizing fatty acid esters of testosterone. McEwen et al. (290) have suggested that di-
hydrotestosterone is the active form of testosterone.
It does appear that testosterone esters are legitimate
pro-drugs of testosterone. However, because the major
evaluation of their release characteristics is based on
some pharmacological effect, some minor doubt does
exist as to whether the esters are truly pro-drugs.
     Junkmann and Witzel (267) document the various
testosterone esters available commercially in Europe.
In the United States, XCII, XCVI, XCVIII and testosterone phenylacetate (C) are all commercially available
as depot forms of testosterone.
     Nandrolone (nortestosterone, CI) and various nan-
drolone derivatives have also been esterified for the
purpose of prolonging the action of these anabolic
agents after their S.C. or I.M. injection in an oil
vehicle (291-295,267,271). Nandrolone phenylpropionate
(CII) and nandrolone decanoate (CIII) are both commercially available. CIII is longer acting than CII and
is administered monthly whereas CIII is administered
weekly (296). The longer activity of CIII (myotrophic
effects as measured by seminal vesicle growth in rats)
with a single 4 mg I.M. dose in sesame oil relative to
CII (similarly administered) was demonstrated by de
Visser and Overbeek (295). The action of CII and the
mechanisms of anabolic androgenic activity were latter
discussed by van der Vies (295). A quantitative structure anabolic activity analysis of a series of nandrolone esters has recently been presented by Chaudry and
James (294) while Pala et al. (291) tested terpenoates

of nandrolone for anabolic activity.

Depot forms (I.M. injection in an oil vehicle) of other steroids are also quite common. The weekly use of dromostanolone propionate in the treatment of breast carcinoma was discussed by Seay et al. (297). Long acting estrogenic steroids useful in the treatment of estrogen deficiency in women has been a goal of many workers. Derivatives of estradiol (CIV), such as the oligemeric derivatives (CV longest acting derivative) of Kuhl et al. (298), polyestradiol phosphate (CVI) of Diczfalusy et al. (299), estradiol 3-benzoate-17-cyclooctenyl ether (CVII) of Falconi et al. (300), 3- and/or 17-acyl derivatives of estradiol of Ferrin (301), and others (302-310) were all shown to have prolonged estrogenic action on I.M. administration. CVI was also found to be useful in the treatment of prostatic carcinoma. Prolonged release forms of dihydroxy progesterone for birth control (acetophenide derivatives) have been found useful (311-313) while the caproate ester of hydroxyprogesterone (Delalutin®) is used as a long acting steroid in amonorrhea (314).

The use of desoxycorticosterone acetate and trimethylacetate in adrenal insufficiency (Addison's disease) has proven successful (315). Desoxycorticosterone trimethylacetate (CIX, Percorten® pivalate) has a very prolonged action and should not be administered more than once a month (316).

Long acting, pro-drug repository injectable forms of corticosteroids useful in the treatment of inflammation are betamethasone acetate, methylprednisolone acetate (Depo-Medrol®), fluorocortisone acetate (Florinef® acetate), hydrocortisone cypionate (Cortef®) and triamcinolone hexacetonide (Aristocort®), to name a few (316).

Winter et al. (317) found that the release of the parent steroid into general circulation was a function not only of the physical properties of the pro-drug (affecting the release from the injection site) but also the chemical properties of the pro-drug (affecting the regeneration rate of steroid once released from the injection site).

Fluphenazine (CX) dihydrochloride is a drug useful in the control of psychotic behavior and is administered orally or by I.M. injection (318). Patient compliance with antipsychotic drugs is a real problem (319). Fluphenazine enanthate (CXI) and fluphenazine decanoate (CXII) are fluphenazine esters given by I.M. injection (in sesame oil vehicle) which have prolonged activity for up to two and four weeks (318,320-324).

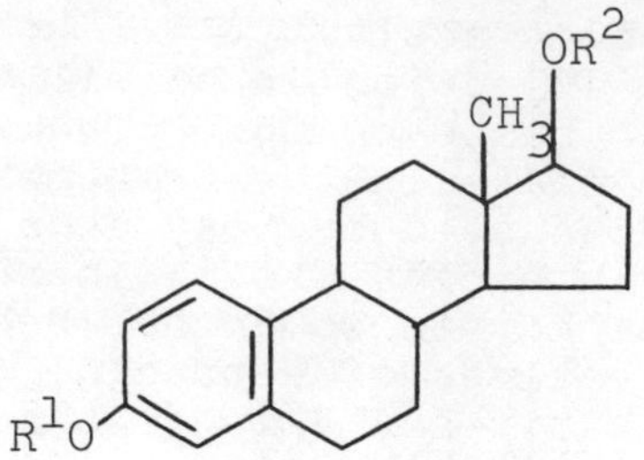

(CIV): $R^1 = R^2 = -H$

(CVII): $R^1 = -COC_6H_5$, $R^2 = $

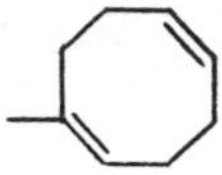

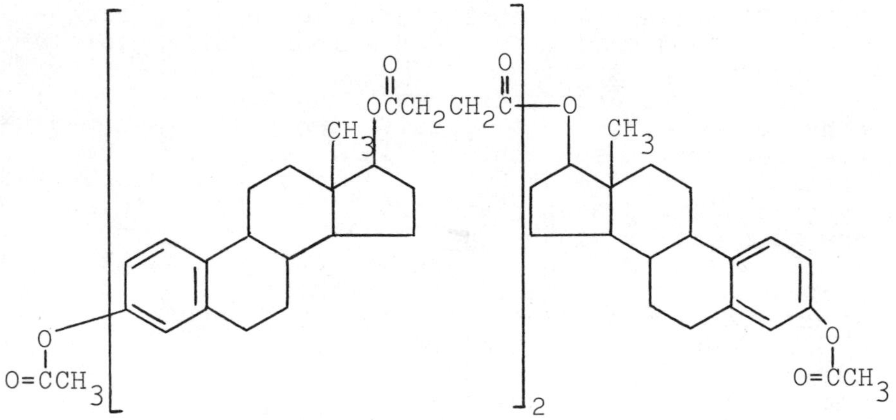

(CV)

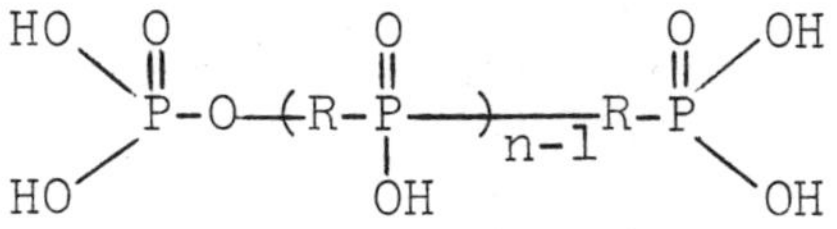

(CVI): R = estradiol
molecule

Depot forms of other neuroleptic drugs effected by esterification (325-331) and I.M. dosing in an oil vehicle are α-fluphenthixol (CXIII), as its decanoate ester
(CXIV), and pipothiazine (CXV) as its palmitate (CXVI)
and undecanoate esters (CXVII).

The prolongation of neuroleptic activity of CXIV
in Viscoleo® administered I.M. compared to CXIII dihydrochloride was demonstrated by Nymark et al. (325).
Figure 7 compares the inhibition of a conditional

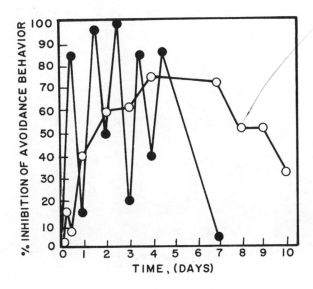

Acta Pharmacologica et Toxicologica

*Figure 7. Days after drug administration—single I.M.
dose of CXIV in oil (◯) or CXIII oral daily (●) (325)*

avoidance response after oral CXIII dihydrochloride
administered once daily (5 mg/Kg) to CXIV (10 mg/Kg)
after a single I.M. injection in oil. Dreyfus et al.
(323) in the case of CX esters, Villeneuve et al. (327)
in the case of CXV esters, and Jorgensen et al. (326)
in the case of CXIII esters were able to show that the
metabolic pattern of the esters was identical to those

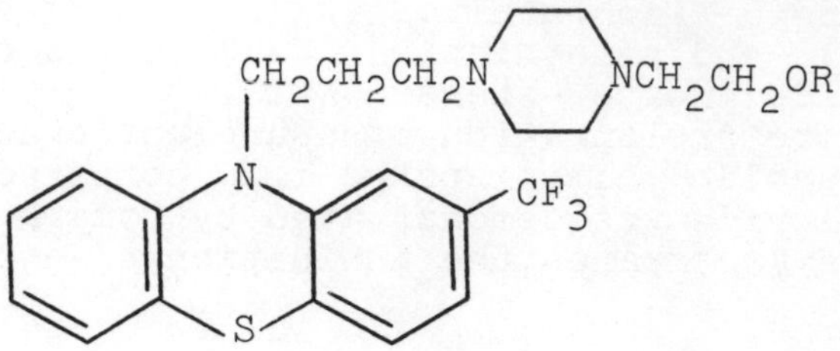

(CX): R = -H

(CXI): R = $-COC_6H_{13}$

(CXII): R = $-COC_9H_{19}$

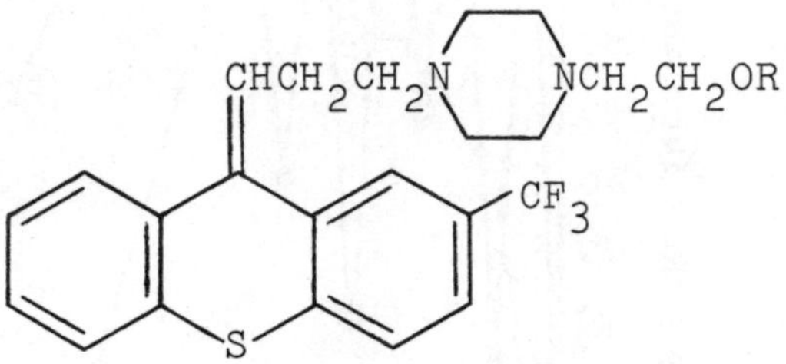

(CXIII): R = -H

(CXIV): R = $-COC_9H_{19}$

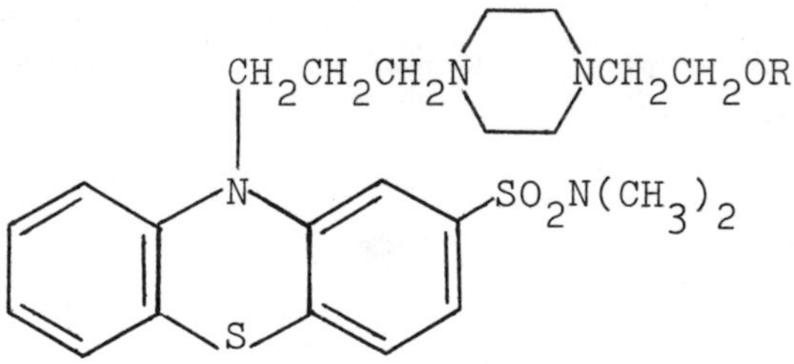

(CXV): R = -H

(CXVI): R = $-COC_{15}H_{31}$

(CXVII): R = $-COC_{10}H_{21}$

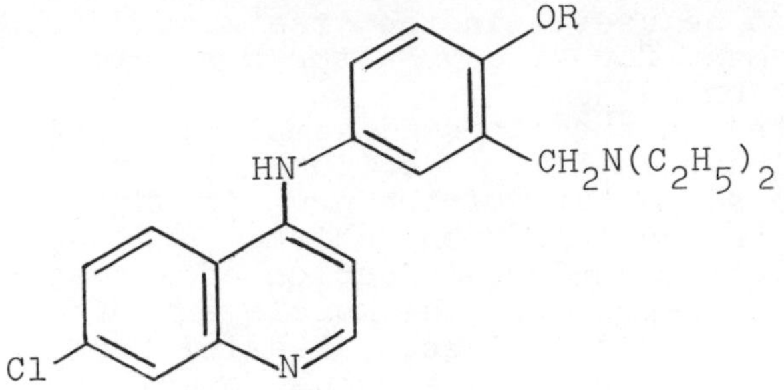

(CXIX):   R = -H
(CXX):   R = -COC$_{15}$H$_{31}$

of the parent compounds and that the activity of the esters appeared to be related to the formation of the parent neuroleptic.

Another parenteral repository pro-drug effected through ester formation was O-palmitoylamodiaquine (CXX), a moderately successful depot form of amodiaquine (CXIX) (332). Elslager (333), in his review of chemotherapy in the treatment of malaria and in particular repository forms of antimalarial drugs, discussed at great lengths various means by which the duration of action of various antimalarial agents could be extended. The two most interesting examples given were various acylated and Schiff base forms of 4,4'-diaminodiphenylsulfone (LXXXVIII) and the use of sparingly water soluble salts of cycloguanil (CXXI) and chloroguanide (CXXII).

4,4'-Diacetoamidodiphenylsulfone (CXXIII) was found to give a repository antimalarial effect when injected I.M. to P. berghei infected mice. However, CXXIII had poor activity in rats. The poor activity in rats was attributed by Thompson (334) to the inability of rats to metabolize CXXIII to LXXXVIII whereas

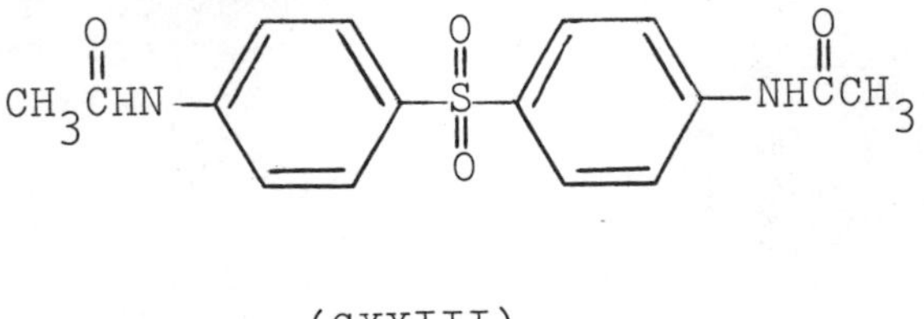

(CXXIII)

mice were able to convert CXXIII to LXXXVIII. CXXIII
was found to be useful in the treatment of P. falici-
parum in humans for 42 days after a single 3.25 mg/Kg
I.M. injection (333).

     As noted in the steroid examples, the ability of
a drug to leave an I.M. injection site is highly dependent on the solubility of the drug in physiological
fluids and in the injection vehicle. If the drug is
water insoluble, an I.M. injection of a suspension of
the drug will deposit in the muscle and over a period
of time gradually dissolves, releasing the drug into
general circulation. The aqueous solubility of any
amine salt is dependent on the counter anion with the
solubility equal to the square root of the solubility
product of the salt. The solubility and stability of
the salt is highly pH dependent.

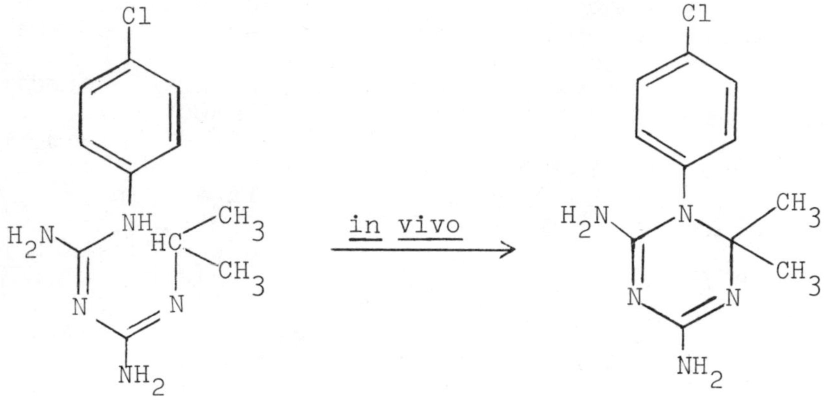

(CXXII)   (CXXI)

     The poor in vitro activity of chloroguanide
(CXXII) compared to its good in vivo activity suggested
that CXXII was metabolized in the body to an active
metabolite (335-340). This active metabolite was found
to be cycloguanil (CXXI) which has a short duration of
action because of rapid excretion (333). Various sparingly water soluble salts of CXXII were found to be
poor repository forms of CXXII but the pamoate salt of
CXXI (CXXIV) with an aqueous solubility of 0.03 mg/ml
at pH 7 was found to be effective against P. berghei in
infected mice for up to 8 1/2 weeks when given S.C.

(<u>333</u>). Figure 8 shows a plot of the logarithm PMW,
the estimated weeks 50% of the mice were protected from
challenge with <u>P</u>. <u>berghei</u>, against logarithm S, the
solubility of various salts of CXXI. The solid line is

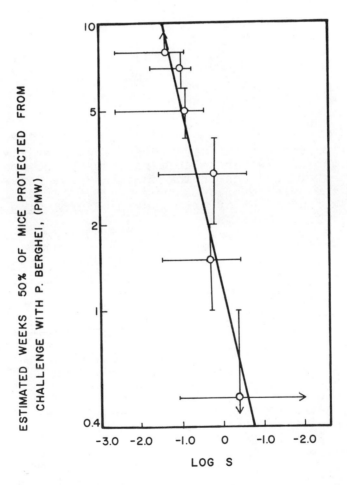

*Figure 8.   Plot of log PMW vs. log (solubility) for a series of
CXXI salts. Plotted from the data of Elslager (333).*

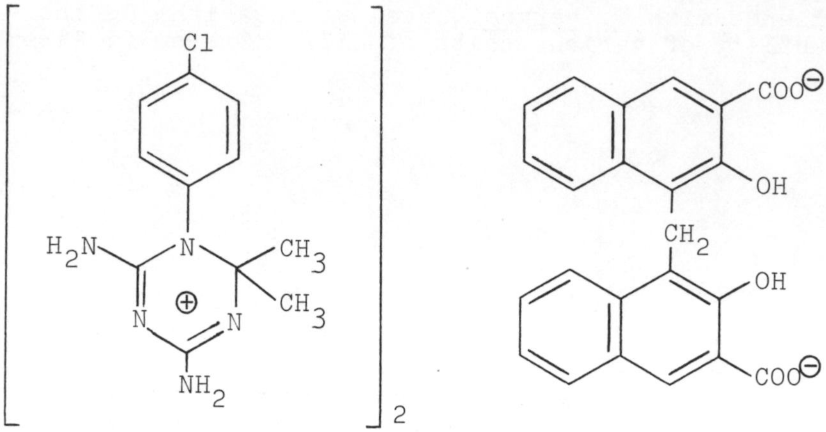

(CXXIV)

the least squares line described by equation 1. The

$$\log PMW = -0.71 \pm 0.11 \log S + 0.077 \underline{\hspace{1cm}} \quad (eq. 1)$$

correlation coefficient was 0.906. As is readily apparent, the less water soluble salts gave the greater
repository effects confirming that the rate determining
step in the release of CXXI from the S.C. injection of
400 mg/Kg equivalent of CXXI was the dissolution of the
sparingly soluble salts.

For a comprehensive review of repository salt, ester and amide forms of various other antimalarials, the
reader is directed to the review by Elslager (333), a
series of papers by Elslager et al. (332,341-344), and
the references therein.

Recently naloxone (CXXV), used as a narcotic antagonist, was found to be very potent but effective for
only three to four hours if administered parenterally
(238-241). Levine et al. (346) found that by giving
I.M. injections of a suspension of naloxone pamoate
(CXXVI) a sustained release action was seen which
blocked the effect of opiates without harmful side effects for up to 72 hours. Use of sparingly soluble
acid salts to effect sustained release after I.M. parenteral administration with a number of other amines
such as streptomycin (347,348) dihydrostreptomycin
(347), naltrexone (349), cyclazocine (350), and others
(351) have proven to be rather successful. Thompson
and Hecht (352) prepared and demonstrated the sustained

release of cyanocobalamine (CXXVII) or vitamin B_{12} from
cyanocobolamine zinc tannate (CXXVIII). Figure 9 shows
the serum levels of CXXVII after I.M. injection of 500
µg of CXXVII in normal saline compared to serum levels
of CXXVII from a molar equivalent amount of CXXVIII.

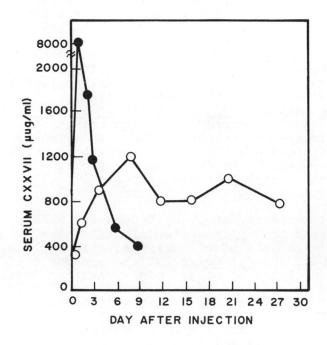

American Journal of Clinical Nutrition

Figure 9.   *CXXVII serum levels in humans after I.M in-*
jection of 500 mg of CXXVII (●) and a molar equivalent
amount of CXXVIII (○) (352)

Parenterally sustained release of acid substances
such as penicillin has similarly been effected by the
use of sparingly soluble salts of penicillin such as
benzathine and procaine penicillin (7-11). The spar-

ingly soluble protamine zinc insulin might also be considered as a chemical modification useful in effecting
sustained release (353) of insulin.

Attempts to produce sustained release or prolonged
action medication for oral administration by the use of
sparingly water soluble salts have been marginally successful. Quinidine polygalacturonate does produce a
prolonged release quinidine on oral administration
(345). The marginal success of these types of products
stems from the fact that the minimum solubility (or
maximum stability) of the salts occurs around neutral-
ity. Because the GI tract has a wide spectrum of pH
(from the strong acid of the stomach to the slightly
alkaline lower intestine), many of the complex salts
(including resins) tend to dissociate and dissolve more
rapidly than the equilibrium solubility of the salts
(or resins) might indicate. Marginal prolonged release
effects were noted with codeine resinate (354) and amphetamine resinate (355). Miller et al. (356) in a
clinical study appeared to confirm that a single 75 mg
dose of imipramine pamoate was therapeutically equivalent to divided doses of 25 mg three times a day of
imipramine hydrochloride. Other examples are amphetamine tannate (357), pyrantel pamoate (358,359), pamoates
(360), tannates (351) and resinates (361,362) of various
amine drugs.

An interesting study by Loucas and Haddad (363)
demonstrated that pilocarpine alginate, a sparingly
water soluble salt of pilocarpine, when applied as solid flakes to the cul-de-sac of the eye could effect the
prolonged release of pilocarpine. Another interesting
prolonged release pro-drug is triacetin (CXXIX), a dermal delivery form of the fungistatic agent acetic acid
(364). The direct percutaneous application of acetic
acid is too corrosive and short acting while CXXIX
gradually releases acetic acid in noncorrosive quantities. Dimethylol urea (CXXX) and 3-methylol-5,5-di-
methylhydantoin (CXXXI) are two prolonged release forms
of the skin disinfectant formaldehyde (CXXXII). Both
drugs, when applied dermally, gradually release CXXXII
(364,365).

The use of polyethylene glycol derivatives
(CXXXIII) of procaine (CXXXIV) by Weiner and Zilkha
(366) to prolong the local anesthetic action of dermally applied procaine was successful. CXXXIII and the
equivalent derivative with PEG 400 showed a slower onset of action but an increase in duration of action.
The results were consistent with CXXXIV being the active agent rather than the intact CXXXIII.

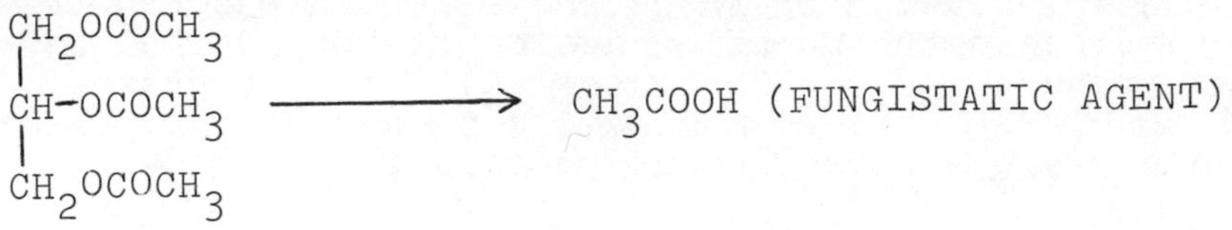

$$CH_2OCOCH_3$$
$$\mid$$
$$CH-OCOCH_3 \longrightarrow CH_3COOH \text{ (FUNGISTATIC AGENT)}$$
$$\mid$$
$$CH_2OCOCH_3$$

(CXXIX)

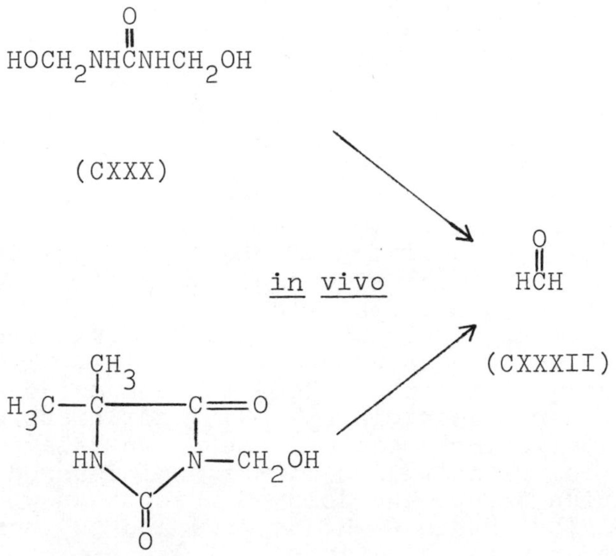

$$\overset{\displaystyle O}{\overset{\displaystyle \|}{HOCH_2NHCNHCH_2OH}}$$

(CXXX)

in vivo

$$\overset{\displaystyle O}{\overset{\displaystyle \|}{HCH}}$$

(CXXXII)

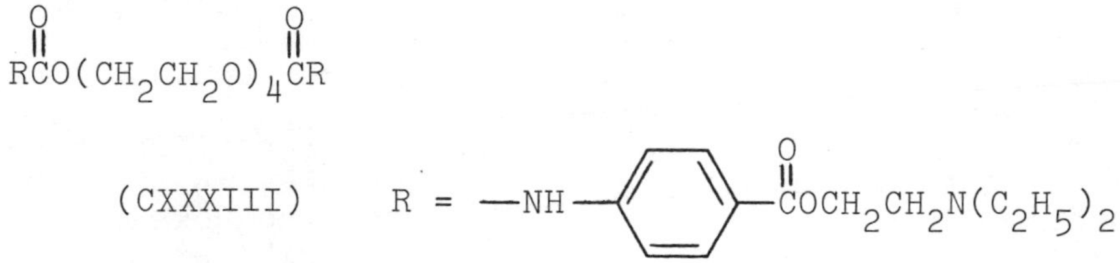

$$H_3C-\overset{\displaystyle CH_3}{\overset{\displaystyle |}{C}}-C=O$$
$$HN \qquad N-CH_2OH$$
$$C$$
$$\|$$
$$O$$

(CXXXI)

$$\overset{\displaystyle O}{\overset{\displaystyle \|}{RCO}}(CH_2CH_2O)_4\overset{\displaystyle O}{\overset{\displaystyle \|}{CR}}$$

(CXXXIII) $R = -NH-\langle\text{C}_6\text{H}_4\rangle-\overset{\displaystyle O}{\overset{\displaystyle \|}{C}}OCH_2CH_2N(C_2H_5)_2$

$$(H_5C_2)_2NCH_2CH_2O\overset{\displaystyle O}{\overset{\displaystyle \|}{C}}-\langle\text{C}_6\text{H}_4\rangle-NH_2$$

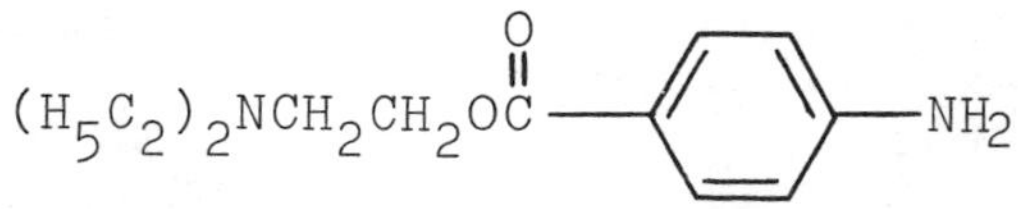

(CXXXIV)

Esterification of insect repellent dihydroxyace-
tone increased the duration action of this dermally applied product (367). Garner et al. (367) suggested
that the intact esters may have some activity of their
own and may not be acting as pro-drugs.

The Use of Pro-Drugs to Increase the Aqueous Solubility of a Drug to Allow for Either Direct Aqueous I.V. or I.M. Injection, or Opthalmic Delivery

As we have already seen, many drugs possess very
poor aqueous solubility which often leads to limited
oral bioavailability. Similarly, many drugs on oral
dosing undergo "first pass" metabolism. Parenteral administration of drugs as aqueous solutions either intravenously or intramuscularly has many advantages:
(a) allows rapid blood levels of the drug to be obtained. This is especially useful in emergency treat-
ments; (b) efficient delivery of the drug, especially
for drug testing; and (c) allows delivery of a drug
when oral therapy is not feasible.
A number of sparingly water soluble drugs are administered in mixed organic/aqueous vehicles. I.M. injections of chlordiazepoxide (368), diazepam (369-370),
and sodium diphenylhydantoin (371-375) administered in
propylene glycol/water vehicles have shown delayed absorption due to precipitation of the administered drug
at the injection site. The delayed absorption with
sodium diphenylhydantoin (I.M. dosing) led to increased
seizure rates in treated patients (374).
As discussed earlier, steroids are a group of compounds with poor aqueous solubility. Adrenal corticosteroids such as betamethasone, dexamethasone, hydrocortisone, methylprednisolone and prednisolone are all
available commercially as water soluble sodium phosphate esters or sodium hemisuccinate esters. These
soluble corticosteroids are used in emergency treatment
of bronchial asthma (status asthmaticus), acute adrenal
cortical insufficiency, allergic drug reactions and are
given intraarticularly or intrasynovially in the treatment of joint inflammation. The water soluble pro-
drugs (CXXXV as sodium phosphate, or CXXXVI as sodium
succinate) regenerate the parent steroid in vivo (379).
CXXXV regenerates the parent steroid via acid and alkaline phosphatase enzymes while CXXXVI regenerates the
parent steroid via esterase enzymes.
Lange and Stein (376) synthesized other water soluble derivatives of steroids such as amino acid carbamates (CXXXVII). However, these derivatives were found
to be either inactive or poorly active.

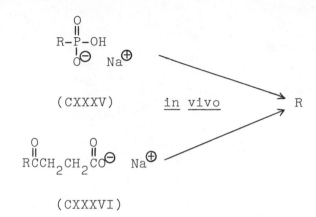

(CXXXV)   in vivo   R

(CXXXVI)

where R = corticosteroid molecule

Although prednisolone hemisuccinate sodium salt
(CXXXIX) is the current commercially available water
soluble form of prednisolone (CXXXVIII), other water
soluble derivatives such as prednisolone-21-m-sulfoben-
zoate sodium salt (XCLI) and prednisolone-21-disodium
phosphate (XCL) have also been synthesized and tested
(377-379). Similarly, methylprednisolone sodium succinate (316,380), hydrocortisone-21-phosphate (379,381),
-21-succinate (316,379,381-382), -21-aminoalkylcarboxy-
lates (383), -21-m-sulfobenzoates (384), and -21-sul-
fates (384), dexamethasone sodium phosphate (316,379),
betamethasone disodium phosphate (316) have been synthesized and found to be water soluble, parenterally
bioavailable forms of the parent steroids.

The succinate esters of the various steroids are
useful but suffer somewhat from stability problems,
i.e., the drug must be supplied as a lyophilized powder
for reconstitution (316). Flynn et al. (385), in dis-
cussing the solvolysis and factors affecting the stability of corticosteroid-21-phosphate esters, states
that "additionally, some types of phosphate esters are
sufficiently stable to allow the formulation of solutions with practical shelf-lives." Another added advantage of phosphate esters as opposed to the succinate
esters is their very rapid conversion to the parent
steroid. Melby et al. (379) in a very interesting
study showed that I.M. administered hydrocortisone-21-
phosphate (XCLII), (XCL), dexamethasone-21-phosphate
(XCLIII) and I.V. administered XCLII all produced
higher plasma levels of the parent steroid than the
corresponding 21-succinate esters. (see Figure 10).

$$\overset{O}{\overset{\|}{RC}}NHCH_2\overset{O}{\overset{\|}{C}}O^{\ominus} \quad K^{\oplus}$$

(CXXXVII):   R = various steroid molecules

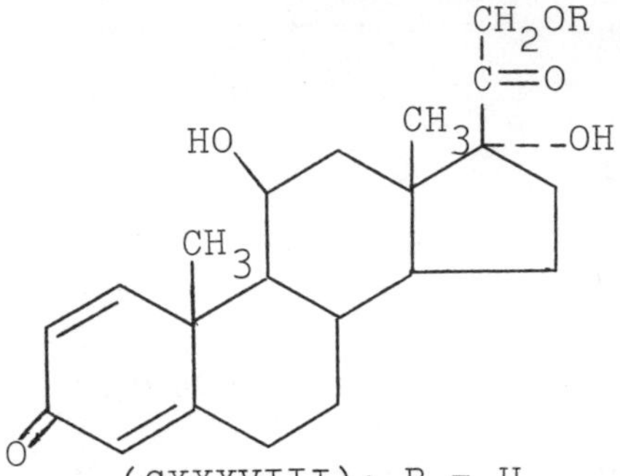

(CXXXVIII): R = H

(CXXXIX): R = $-COCH_2CH_2COO^{\ominus}$ $Na^{\oplus}$

(XCL): R = $-PO_3^{\ominus}$ x $2Na^{\oplus}$

(XCLI): R = $-CO-\langle\!\langle\rangle\!\rangle$ $SO_3^{\ominus}$ $Na^{\oplus}$

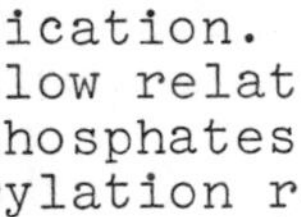

It was suggested by Melby et al. (379) that the 21-suc-
cinate esters underwent metabolism at other points in
the molecule before de-esterification. This could occur if de-esterification was slow relative to other
metabolic processes. The 21-phosphates, on the other
hand, undergo rapid dephosphorylation releasing the
parent steroid. Although Melby et al.'s (379) data
does not suggest it, another possible mechanism is that
the 21-succinate might be excreted unchanged. The active elimination of acidic drugs such as penicillin and
probenicid have been shown to occur (386).
     Sandman et al. (387,388) in studying the aqueous
stability of chloramphenicol succinate (XCLIV), a water
soluble pro-drug of chloramphenicol (XCLV) suitable for
I.V., I.M. and opthalmic delivery of chloramphenicol,
noted an unusual partial acyl transfer reaction (see
scheme IX) of the succinyl group to give a cyclic hemi-
ortho ester (XCLVI). A similar reaction may also potentially occur for hydrocortisone (see Scheme X).

XCLIX, if formed, would be more stable, i.e., would not be subjected to esterase activity, and might be eliminated or metabolized via other pathways.

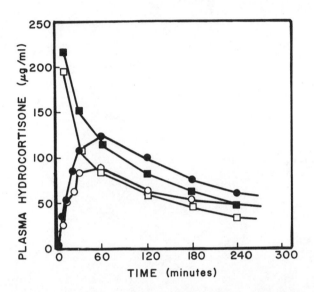

Metabolism

Figure 10. Mean 17,21-dihydroxy-20-oxosteroids in plasma following I.M. injection of XCLII (●), I.V. injection of XCLII (■), I.M. injection of hydrocortisone-21-succinate (○), and I.V. injection of hydrocortisone-21-succinate (□), in a dose of 1mg/kg of body weight in humans (379)

The estrogenic steroid, diethylstilbesterol (CL), may be given I.V. as its diphosphate ester (CLI) disodium salt in the treatment of prostatic carcinoma. However, the original synthesis of CLI was not done with the intention of obtaining a water soluble form of CL but to help localize CL in the carcinoma cells by utilizing the high acid and alkaline phosphatase levels (389-397) in carcinoma cells to effect preferential uptake of CL. Water soluble glycine esters of CL have

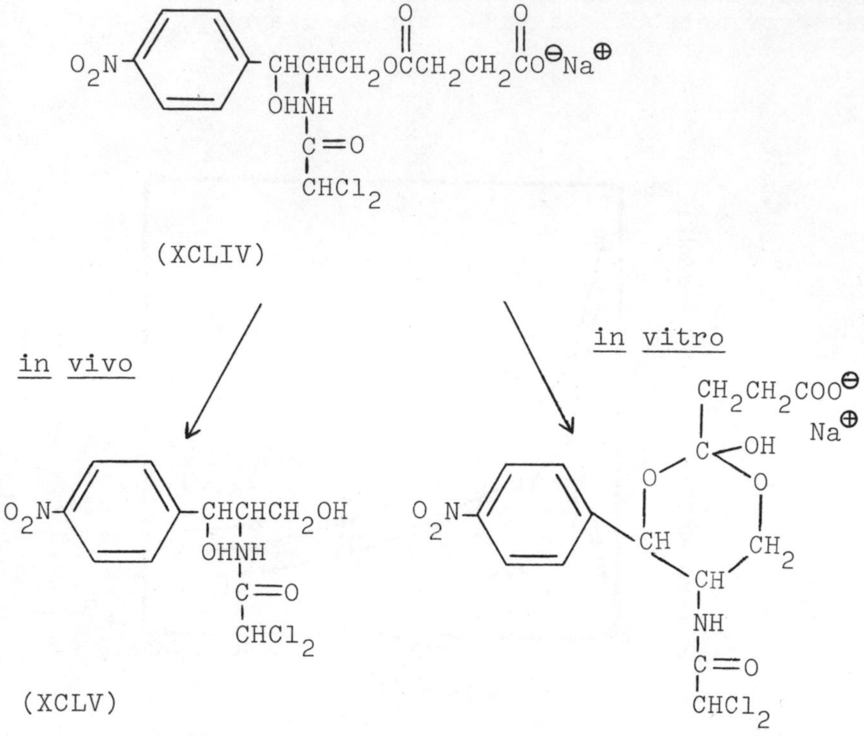

(XCLIV)

in vivo   in vitro

(XCLV)   (XCLVI)

Scheme IX

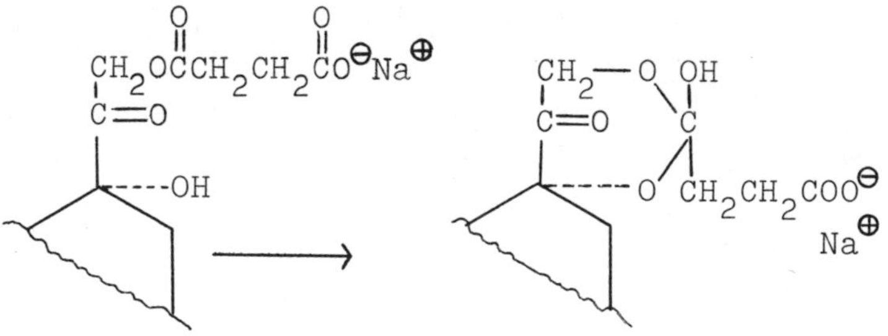

(XCLVIII)   (XCLIX)

Scheme X

also been synthesized (398).

Hydroxydione (CLII) is a water insoluble basal anesthetic that may be given I.V. (398) as its sodium succinate derivative (CLIII).

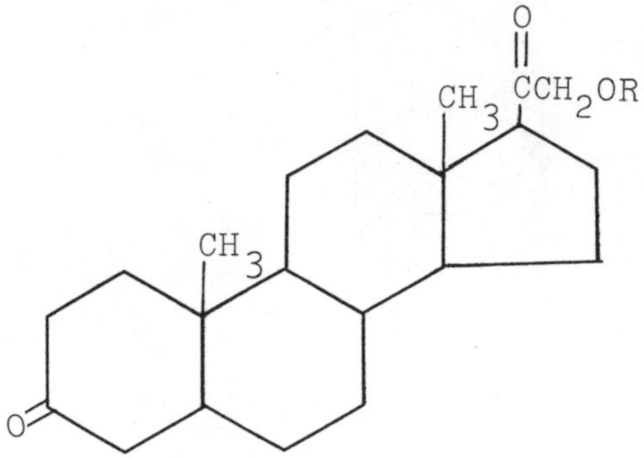

$$(CLII): \quad R = -H$$
$$(CLIII): \quad R = -COCH_2CH_2COO^{\ominus}Na^{\oplus}$$

As stated earlier, chloramphenicol (XCLV), a slightly water soluble antibiotic, cannot be used directly for I.V., or I.M. injection or for local solution application as eye/ear drops. Glazko et al. (399) overcame this problem by synthesizing the sodium salt of chloramphenicol monosuccinate (XCLIV). XCLIV can be given I.V./I.M. as a reconstituted injectable and is reasonably quantitavely converted to XCLV and succinic acid (399) by esterase activity present in plasma (400-402). Adenine arabinoside (CLIV), an antiviral, cytotoxic agent whose low aqueous solubility prevented its use in small volume I.V. preparations, was solubilized by preparation of the 5'-formate ester (CLV) (see paper by Dr. Repta). LePage et al. (403) prepared the 5'-phosphate (CLVI) of CLIV. However, CLVI may undergo deamination before regenerating CLIV which may limit its usefulness (403,404).

Oxazepam (CLVII), a minor tranquilizer and actually a metabolite of diazepam (405-408), has been solubilized as oxazepam sodium succinate (CLVIII). CLVIII is a pro-drug of CLVII with favorable physical properties for I.V. or I.M. administration (409-413). An interesting side line to this work is that the number 3 carbon of CLVII is an optically active center and the two possible isomers of CLVIII have been shown to regenerate CLVII at differing rates (410). The dif-

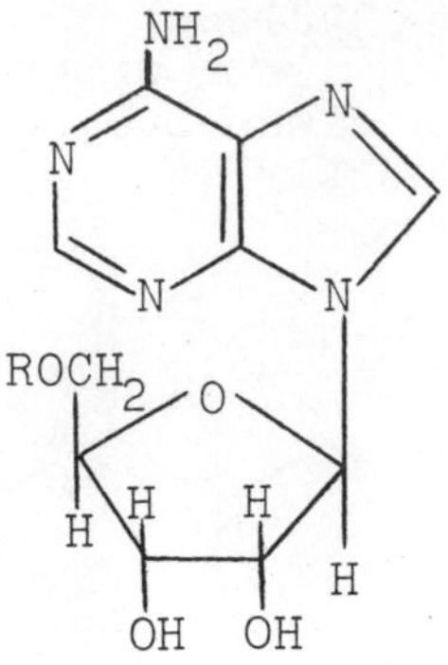

(CLIV): R = -H

(CLV): R = -COH

(CLVI): R = -PO$_3$H$^{\ominus}$Na$^{\oplus}$

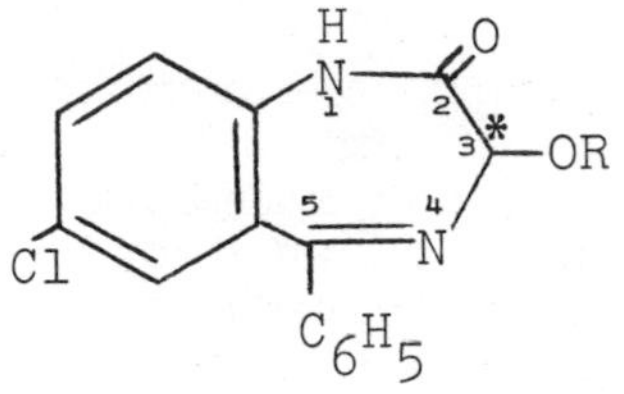

(CLVII): R = -H

(CLVIII): R = -COCH$_2$CH$_2$COO$^{\ominus}$Na$^{\oplus}$

fering rates were also found to be a function of the
particular animal species in which the regeneration was
studied (410).

Recently Stella and Higuchi (414) synthesized and
demonstrated the possible usefulness of β,N',N'-diethyl-
aminoethyl-5-methyl-2,2-ethylphenylhydantoate (CLIX)
as a water soluble pro-drug of mephenytoin (CLX).
CLIX is converted to CLX under physiological conditions
without enzyme mediation. Currently the only injectable anticonvulsant hydantoin available is sodium diphenylhydantoin which, due to its alkalinity, has many
unwanted side effects (415). A derivative of 5,5-di-
phenylhydantoin similar to CLIX will be reported by
Stella et al. later.

Bioreversible chemical modification of drug molecules to increase the aqueous solubility of a compound
has also been utilized in solubilizing menadione,
either as its bisulfite adduct, its disodium diphosphate ester, or its carboxymethoxime derivative (416-
418), tetrahydrocannabinol as a series of bifunctional
esters (419-421), and α-methydopa as its ethyl ester
(422).

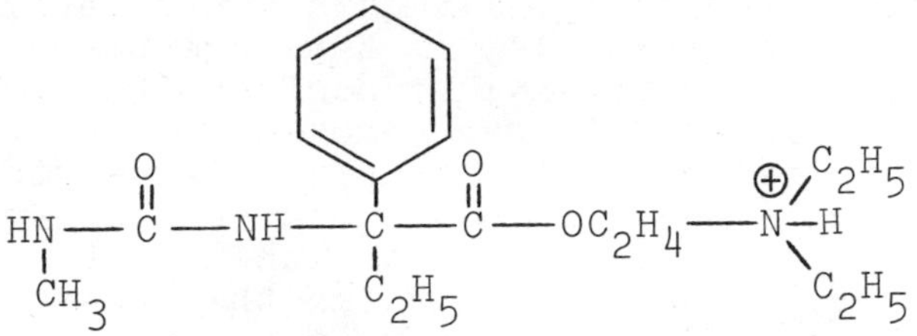

$$HN-\overset{\overset{O}{\|}}{C}-NH-\overset{\underset{CH_3}{|}}{\underset{}{C}}... $$

(CLIX)

in vivo/in vitro

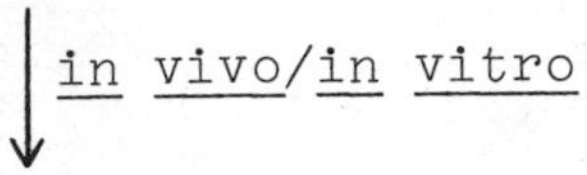

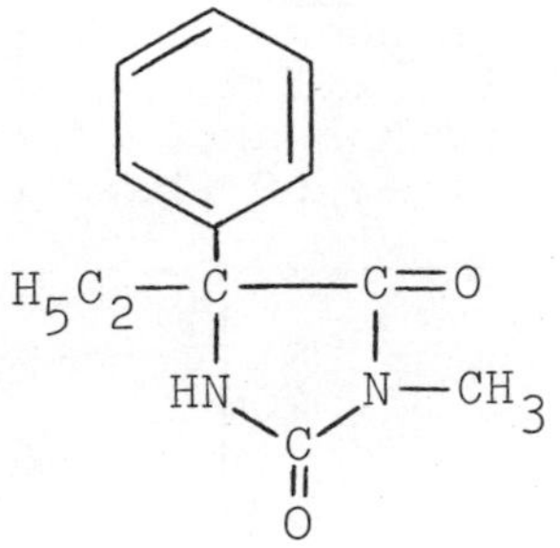

(CLX)

The Use of Pro-Drugs to Lower the Toxicity of a Drug

A drug may exhibit toxicity if it accumulates
selectively in some tissue or organ and interacts with
some receptor in the organ thus eliciting a reaction
which is not necessarily the desired pharmacological
reaction. Any drug-receptor interaction will be dependent on the amount of drug reaching the receptor and
its time profile in contact with the receptor. As
stated earlier, "peak" and "valley" effects of multiple
dosing might raise the concentration of a drug in the
plasma above its toxic level or, at the end of its

cycle (before the next dose is given), the plasma level
may drop below the therapeutic level. For these reasons, a sustained release or prolonged release form of
a drug may be desirable to narrow the difference seen
between the "peaks" and "valleys." If a pro-drug with
intrinsically lower toxicity is designed to regenerate
the parent compound slowly (the equivalent to slow absorption) the toxicity of the parent compound might be
lowered.

A few interesting, although controversial, and
perhaps marginal examples of this phenomena do exist.
The agent 5,5-ethylphenylhydantoin (CLXI), was used as
an anticonvulsant. It was removed from the market because of toxicity and in its place mephenytoin (CLX)
was promoted (423). It has since been shown that CLX
is N-demethylated to CLXI and although CLX is not without toxicity it is still used in the treatment of petit
mal seizures (423). The known activity of CLX, which
does not involve any lag time, is consistent with CLX
maintaining some anticonvulsant activity of its own.

Similarly primacolone (primidone, CLXII) was promoted as a nontoxic anticonvulsant useful in the treatment of grand mal seizures (424). Specifically, it was
felt that it might replace phenobarbitone (CLXIII). It
has since been found that CLXII is metabolically oxidized to CLXIII both in humans and animals (426-428).
Kutt (425) in a recent review of pharmacodynamic and

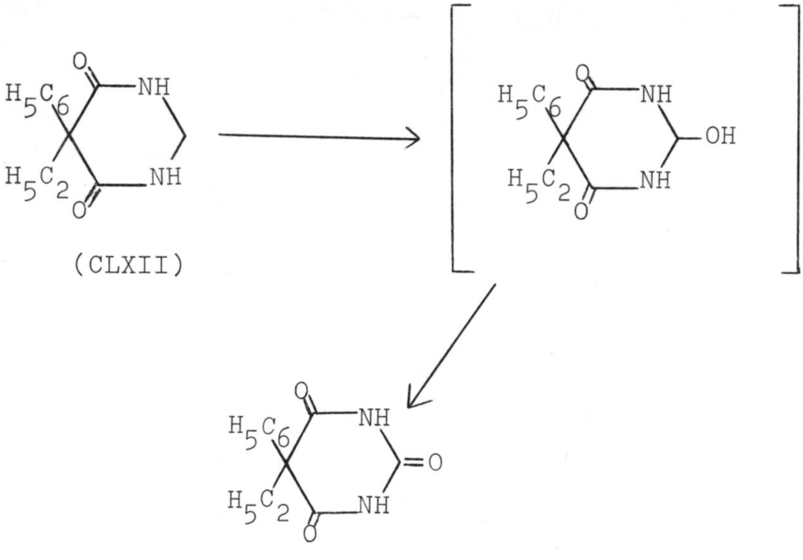

(CLXII)

(CLXIII)

pharmacokinetic measurements of antiepileptic drugs
states that CLXIII plasma levels after chronic administration of CLXII are 1.5-3 times higher than the
CLXII levels. This is consistent with the slow elimination of CLXIII. Even though the long term antiepileptic effects of CLXII might be attributed to its
metabolite, CLXIII, it does appear that CLXII and another metabolite phenylethylmalonamide have anitepilep-
tic activity of their own (425).

Another drug whose toxicity appears related to its
tissue distribution is the cytotoxic agent adriamycin
(CLXIV). The cardiotoxicity of CLXIV has been well established. Arcamone et al. (429) synthesized and
showed the change in CLXIV distribution in mice heart
tissue after the administration of adriamycin-14-oc-
tanoate (CLXV). CLXV was shown to have comparable
cytoxic activity to CLXIV. After CLXV dosing of tri-
tium labelled compound, CLXV showed greater amounts of
radiolabelled material in lungs, liver, and spleen
relative to CLXIV dosed animals, but lower amounts of
radiolabelled materials were seen in the heart and
kidney.

Probably the area of drug toxicity which has been
given the greatest attention and for which the pro-drug
approach has often been used is gastric irritation.
Drug induced gastric ulceration has been a recognized

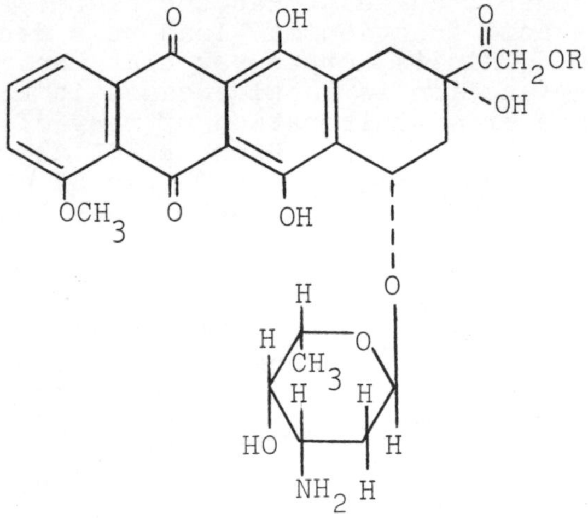

(CLXIV): R = -H

(CLXV): R = -COC$_7$H$_{15}$

problem especially in patients treated for inflammatory
diseases. Salicylates including acetylsalicylic acid
or aspirin, as well as salicylic acid itself, have been
known to induce gastric bleeding, ulceration and general GI irritation (430-441). Attempts to modify salicylic and acetylsalicylic acid irritation by the pro-
drug approach has a long history. None of the products
studied appears to hold any great advantage over acetylsalicylic acid either in activity or decreased gastric irritant properties. However, potential decreased
gastric irritant properties with the use of some of the
pro-drugs have been claimed by some of their promoters
(442-445).

Other salicylic or benzoic acid derivatives which
have shown gastric irritant properties have been chemically modified in attempts to decrease their irritant
properties. The glyceryl ester of N-arylanthranilic
acid apparently has lower gastric irritant properties
than the parent compound (446), while various bioreversible derivatives of nicotinic acid showed no advantage or showed marginal advantages over nicotinic acid
(447-448).

All potent nonsteroidal anti-inflammatory agents
appear to exhibit GI irritant properties. Indomethicin
(CLXVI) has been particularly notorious. The acidic
properties of the anti-inflammatory agents and GI irri-
tants in general suggest that the bioreversible blocking of the acid function may lead to a decrease in GI
irritation. This is not to say that their irritant
mechanism of action is local because it has been shown
that parenteral administration of many of these agents
does promote ulceration. However, it also stands to
reason that high localization in the GI mucosa of these
agents on oral administration can only help promote
rapid ulceration.

Glamkowski et al. (449), although not stating that
their intention was to bypass the gastric irritant
properties of CLXVI, tested the activity of the aldehyde analog of CLXVI. Using the canageenan-induced
foot odema test in the rat, the aldehyde analog (CXVII)
was 0.6-0.7 times as active as CLXVI. Subsequent analysis of plasma showed that CLXVII gave substantial
plasma levels of CLXVI presumably as a result of oxidative metabolism (see Figure 11). Whether the lower
CLXVI levels after CLXVII dosing is due to incomplete
absorption or incomplete metabolism is uncertain. The
authors did not state whether any differences in GI irritant properties between the two compounds existed.

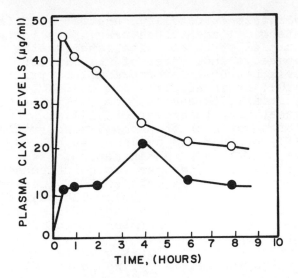

Figure 11. CLXVI plasma level-time profile after administration of CLXVI (○) and CLXVII (●) at a dose of 10 mg/kg orally to rats. Plotted from the data of Glamkowski et al. (449)

(CLXVI): R = —COOH

(CLXVII): R = —COH

Phenylbutazone (CLXVIII), another acid (carbon acid) nonsteroidal agent, has been shown to be a GI irritant. It has yet to be established whether the O-trimethoxybenzoyl enol ester of CLXVIII (CLXIX), which supposedly is better tolerated and less toxic than CLXVIII (450), or an acyclic form of CLXVIII (CLXX), which is partially metabolized to CLXVIII (451-454), hold any great advantage over CLXVIII.

Clofibrate or p-chlorophenoxyisobutyric acid ethyl ester (CLXXI) synthesized by Jones et al. (455) was found to be useful as an antihypercholesteremic agent. It is generally accepted that the corresponding acid, p-chlorophenoxyisobutyric acid (CLXXII), is the pharmacologically active species (456). The use of the ethyl ester as opposed to CLXXII, or one of its salts, appears related to the better tolerance of CLXXI on prolonged administration (457).

Oleandrin, a potent diuretic useful in the treatment of cardiac insufficiency, was esterified to its

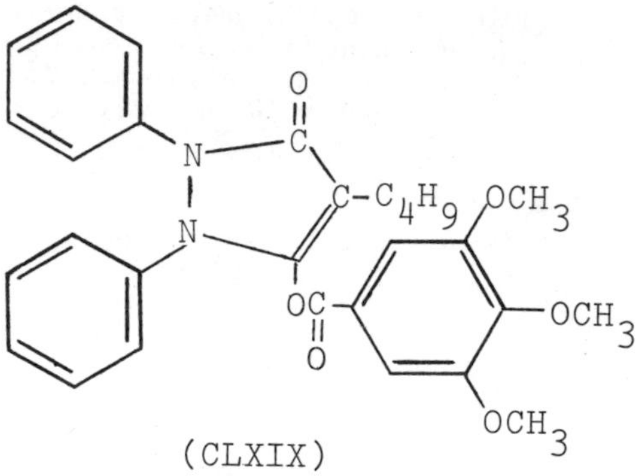

(CLXIX)

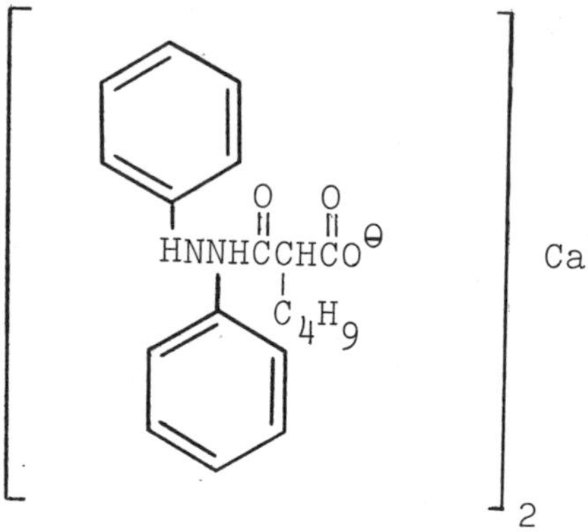

(CLXX)

acetate ester in an attempt to lower its GI distur-
bance tendencies (458-459).

Pain due to I.M. injection is a toxicity problem
that has been associated with a number of compounds.
Intramuscular injections of the antibiotic, clindamycin, were found to be painful but a phosphate ester pro-
drug of clindamycin on I.M. dosing (460-461) was pain-
less. Similarly chloramphenicol sodium succinate (399)
and bioreversible oleandomycin derivatives (168,172-
173) were less irritating on I.M. injection than the
parent compounds.

Subcutaneous and I.M. injection of ionic iron and
colloidal iron were found to be either toxic or very
painful. Martin et al. (462) and others (463-466)
found that iron administered as a dextran iron complex
(Imferon®) was well absorbed after I.M. injection, had
low toxicity and irritation, and was a satisfactory
hematinic agent. Complexes of iron with sorbital (467)
have also proven successful. Terrato et al. (468-470)
have studied oral iron absorption from complexes with
low molecular weight noncarbohydrate polymers and
shown that the absorption is enhanced in the presence
of these chelating agents. In the body, iron is
stored as the complex ferritin and is transported in
combination with the protein β-globulin. The use of
polysaccharide molecules such as dextran, etc., was an
attempt to simulate the naturally occurring macromole-
cules as a transport medium for iron.

Two general examples where the pro-drug approach
has led to a reduction in toxicity but where the mechanisms are not understood are amphotericin methyl ester (CLXXIII) and the ethyl ester of prostaglandin.
Bonner et al. (471) tested both the activity and toxicity of a series of polyene antibiotic esters and found
that the toxicity of the esters was much lower than
the toxicity of the parent compounds. Amphotericin
(CLXXIV) is administered as a large volume I.V. colloid
suspension. The zwitterionic nature of CLXXIV is at-
tested to by its low water solubility at neutral pH
and increasing solubility below pH 2 and above pH 11
(472). CLXXIII is water soluble at neutral pH allowing
it to be administered as true solution. The toxicity
of the original colloidal CLXXIV may have been due to
the I.V. administration of particulate matter. The
activity of CLXXIII versus CLXXIV, against C. albicans
infected mice was essentially identical. The ethyl esters of prostaglandins are claimed by Anderson et al.
(473) to lead to a decrease in diarrhea associated with
prostaglandin administration.

The Use of Pro-Drugs to Overcome Problems of Poor Patient Acceptance of a Product

The commercial potential of a product might be judged in terms of a) its ability to cure or suppress some diseased state more successfully than agents currently available, and b) the potential market produced by that disease. However, a critical consideration often overlooked is a patient acceptance factor. Painful injections might be a deterrent to the use of a drug, especially if multiple dosing is required. An antibiotic might be extremely bitter tasting making it suitable for dosing in a capsule or coated tablet but unsuitable for a pediatric suspension or chewable tablet dosage form. Poor patient acceptance of a product, especially with pediatric and possibly geriatric products, can often be a deterrent factor for commercialization of a product for that segment of the population.

Chloramphenicol (XCLV) is an example of a useful drug which, although sparingly water soluble, had an unpleasant bitter taste. Various derivatives of XCLV such as its palmitate ester (CLXXV) were synthesized and tested for taste acceptance and their ability to deliver XCLV (474-476) on oral dosing. Other sparingly soluble XCLV derivatives have been synthesized in an effort to overcome the taste problem (477-479). Because of the sparingly water soluble nature of CLXXV, it presented a number of oral bioavailability problems that were overcome by the use of a metastable polymorph of CLXXV and the careful screening of particle size effects (480). Glazko et al. (475,481) in their studies of the bioavailability of XCLV from CLXXV noted some unusual results. It might seem that CLXXV should be partially absorbed as such and be converted to XCLV both in the GI tract and plasma but no CLXXV was found in plasma. Recently Andersgaard et al. (482) noted that the dissolution of CLXXV from particles was catalyzed by pancreatic lipase and that on dissolution XCLV was released. Surprisingly the pancreatic lipase did not catalyze the conversion of CLXXV to XCLV in the bulk phase solution. The authors postulate that the pancreatic lipase is actually adsorbed onto the CLXXV particle and actually catalyzes a solid state hydrolysis of the ester to its corresponding acid and alcohol fractions.

A question that probably should be asked is why does a drug taste bitter? Bitterness results from a compound dissolving in the saliva of the mouth and interacting with a bitter taste receptor. Molecular theories on the cause of sweet and bitter taste have appeared in the literature and will not be discussed here (483-485). The general method of overcoming a bitter taste in a pharmaceutical has involved either a formulation technique, i.e. coated tablet, use of capsules, or preparation of a bioreversible, less water soluble derivative of the drug. CLXXV was one example of the latter technique. The lowering of the water solubility does not block the drug-receptor interaction but simply prevents the drug from ever reaching the receptor. If the molecular theory of sweet and bitter receptors is accepted, simply blocking the electrophilic or nucleophilic site of interaction should suffice.

Other examples of pro-drugs used to overcome taste problems are the palmitate ester of clindamycin (to be discussed further by Dr. Sinkula), the stearylsulfate salt of erythromycin (486), the ethylsuccinate and ethyl carbonate esters of erythromycin (178,179), phosphate and carbonate esters of lincomycin (487-489), acyl ester N-oxide oleandomycin (490), and the triacetyl ester of oleandomycin which was less soluble and therefore less bitter than oleandomycin (168,172-173). N'-Acetylsulfisoxazole (Lipogantrisin®) and N'-acetylsulfamethoxypyridazine (Kynex®) were two tasteless derivatives of sulfisoxazole and sulfamethoxypyridazine suitable as pediatric suspensions (491). The 3,4,5-trimethoxybenzoate salt of tetracycline was also found to be tasteless (492).

The unpleasant taste of acetaminophen (CLXXVI) has prevented its use in a chewable tablet formulation for pediatric patients. Repta and Hack (493) prepared 2-(p-acetaminophenoxy)tetrahydropyran (CLXXVII), a prodrug of CLXXVI, which was shown to have a lower water solubility than CLXXVI and is readily converted to CLXXVI under acidic conditions. A series of O-acyl and O-carbonate esters of CLXXVI as pro-drugs of CLXXVI were evaluated by Dittert et al. (494-498). Their objective did not appear to be the blockage of CLXXVI's taste problem. Chloral hydrate (CLXXVIII), a hypnotic, was limited in its use by an unpleasant, bitter taste and odor as well as formulation problems (to be discussed further in the next section). Various derivatives of CLXXVIII have been attempted to overcome the taste and odor problems. One example was dichloralphenazone (CLXXIX), a molecular complex between CLXXVIII and phenazone (499). Alternatively CLXXVIII is considered to be a precursor (a pro-drug) of trichloroethanol (CLXXX), a high boiling point corrosive liquid (500). Solid pro-drugs of CLXXX have been promoted (497,498,501,502), including triclorphos (CLXXXI),

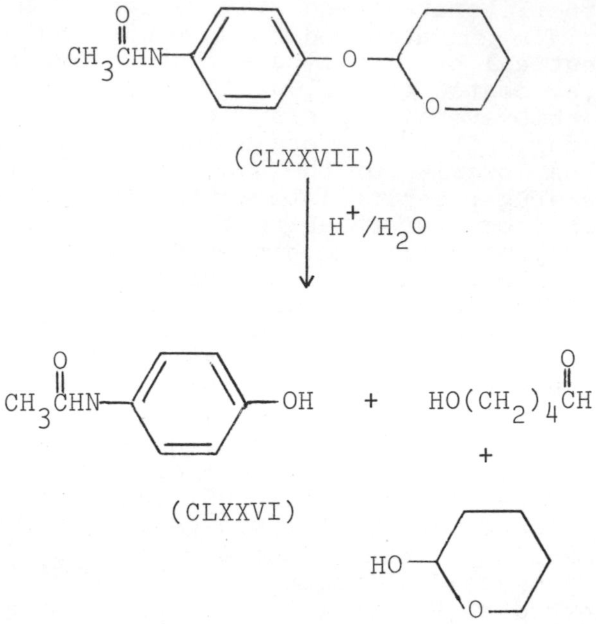

(CLXXVII)

$$H^+/H_2O$$

(CLXXVI)

bis-trichloroethyl carbonate (CLXXXII) and trichloro-
ethyl-4-acetamidophenyl carbonate (CLXXXIII).

Bitterness associated with amine drugs are well
documented (361,362). Borodkin et al. (361,362) prepared a series of slightly soluble ion exchange resinates of a series of amine drugs with the objective of
preparing products suitable for a chewable tablet dosage form. The slightly water soluble pyruvium pamoate
(Povan®) is described as a pleasant tasting suspension
(503) while the tranquilizer/antihistamine hydroxyzine
pamoate (Vistarl®) and the antiemetic diphenidol
pamoate (Vontrol®) are also slightly water soluble
tasteless suspensions (504,505). Similarly the sparingly water soluble napsylate salt of propoxyphene
(Darvon-N®) was promoted as a tasteless and stable derivative of propoxyphene (506,508). Propoxyphene could
not be prepared in a liquid dosage form because of
stability problems or in a pediatric dosage form because of bitterness. Various sulfonic acid salts were
found to be tasteless (506,509) because of their low
aqueous solubility.

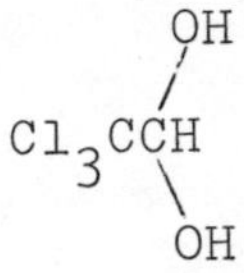

$$Cl_3CCH(OH)_2$$
(with structure: Cl_3CCH bearing two OH groups)

(CLXXVIII)

$$Cl_3CCH_2OH$$

(CLXXX)

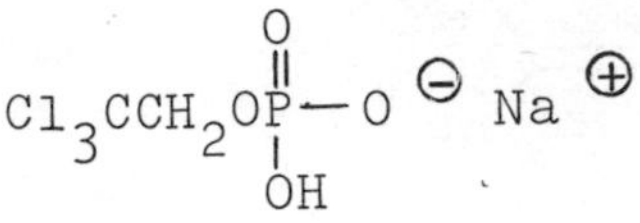

$$Cl_3CCH_2O\overset{O}{\underset{OH}{P}}-O^{\ominus} \ Na^{\oplus}$$

(CLXXXI)

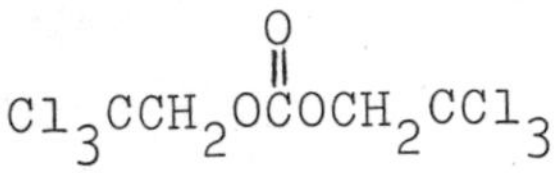

$$Cl_3CCH_2O\overset{O}{\overset{\|}{C}}OCH_2CCl_3$$

(CLXXXII)

$$CH_3\overset{O}{\overset{\|}{C}}HN-\underset{\text{(benzene ring)}}{}-O\overset{O}{\overset{\|}{C}}OCH_2CCl_3$$

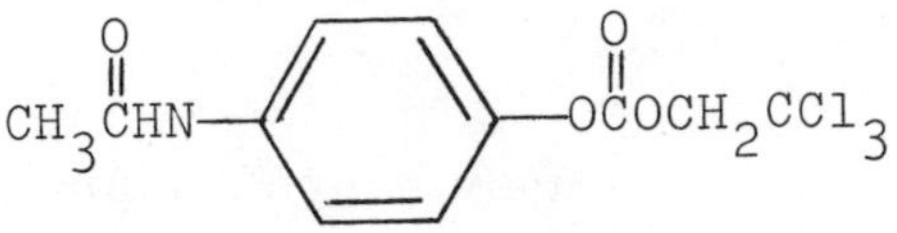

(CLXXXIII)

The Use of Pro-Drugs to Promote Site Specific Delivery of a Drug

Ideally, pro-drugs might be useful in promoting site specificity for a given drug by localizing the drug in a target organ by utilizing either some specific physical or chemical property of the site. For example, tumor cells are postulated to contain a higher concentration of phosphatase and amidase enzymes than normal cells (510). Therefore, if a cytotoxic drug is phosphorylated (assuming a suitable functional group for attachment is available), the tumor cells will provide a "sink" for the drug thus promoting a somewhat specific accumulation of the drug at that site. Phosphoryl derivatives of cytotoxic agents such as diethylstilbesterol (CLXXXIVa and CLXXXIVb) and estradiol (CVI) have been found useful in the treatment of prostatic carcinoma (299,389-397) presumably due to this specificity. Phosphate esters of cytosine arabinoside (511,512) and adenine arabinoside (403,404) have not proven to be any more active than the parent compounds. The dicarbamate of CLXXXIVa, (CLXXXV), has also been suggested for the treatment of prostatic carcinoma (513). The parent compounds in each of these cases are

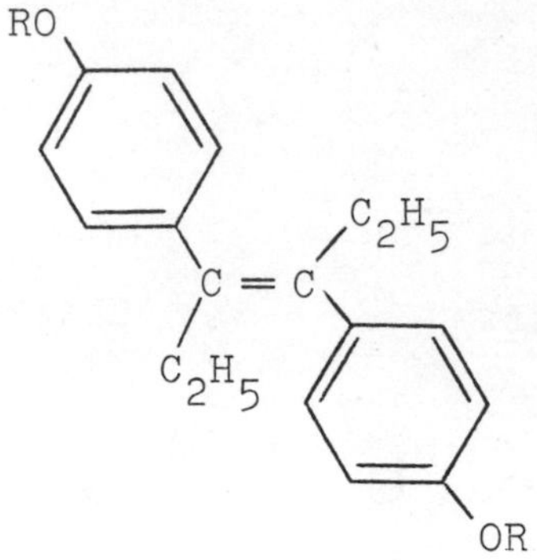

(CLXXXIVa): R = -H(diethylstilbesterol)

(CLXXXIVb): R = $-PO_3H^{\ominus}Na^{\oplus}$

(CLXXXV): R = $-CONH_2$

the active agent with the precursors having little intrinsic activity.

Localization of drugs at a site has received some
success with the bowel sterilants, succinyl and phtha-
loyl sulphathiazole (514). Both these derivatives are
monoamides of sulphathiazole which, due to their polarity, are not well absorbed from the GI tract. In the
lower intestine and colon, both release sulphathiazole
which then acts as the bowel sterilant. Another pro-
drug which has shown some site specificity is oxypheni-
satin and its diacetate derivative (CLXXXVII). CLXXXVI

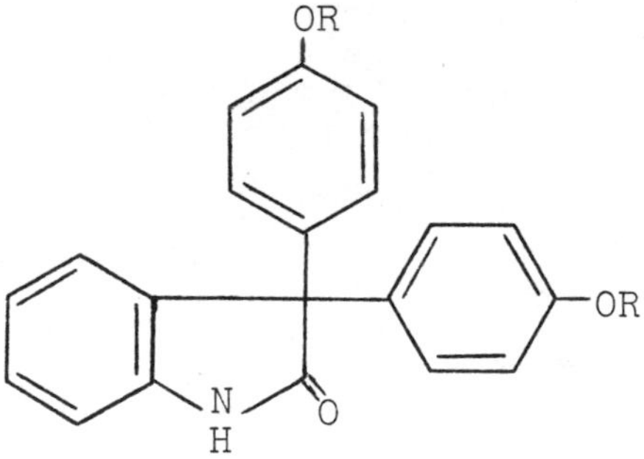

(CLXXXVI): R = -H

(CLXXXVII): R = $-COCH_3$

itself is active as a bowel evacuant if administered
rectally as a solution. CLXXXVII is active orally and
is metabolized to CLXXXVI in the intestines and exerts
its evacuant properties as CLXXXVI. Bruzzese et al.
(515) and Hubacher et al. (516) have surveyed the effect of acetylation of diphenolic laxatives and found
the diacetyl derivatives to be less potent than the dihydroxy metabolite per se. However, the acetylated derivatives are less irritating and more stable when administered orally.

Other examples of site specificity through pro-
drugs were discussed earlier, e.g., promotion of passage through the blood brain barrier and changing the
permeability characteristics of various polar chelating
agents. Methenamine (I), a pro-drug of formaldehyde,
offers site specificity for formaldehyde to the urinary
tract. When administered orally in an enteric coated
tablet, I is absorbed and excreted in the urine. Acid-
ification of the urine by either dietary regulation or
coadministration of acidifying agents such as ammonium
chloride or sodium biphosphate promotes formation of
the nonspecific antibacterial formaldehyde (22). The
enteric coating of methenamine tablets is necessary to
prevent gastric acidity from converting I to formaldehyde prematurely (22).

An example of a product which may be considered a
pro-drug is selenium sulfide. Selenium derivatives are
useful as antiseborrheic and antibacterial agents
(517). However, the more water soluble derivatives are
also toxic due to systemic selenium absorption. Selenium sulfide is a very slightly soluble selenium derivative useful for local application in the treatment of
dandruff. The poor solubility allows for local effect
while preventing systemic toxicity.

The Use of Pro-Drugs to Eliminate Stability and Other Formulation Problems

The stability of a drug in its dosage form, whether a liquid or solid dosage form, can limit the commercial potential of a drug product. Most drug stability
problems can generally be overcome via physical means
rather than chemical means. That is, if a drug, useful
as an injectable, is sparingly stable in aqueous solution, lypophylization of the drug and simple reconstitution with a solvent before administration to the patient might be the answer to the stability problem.

The pro-drug approach has been utilized with vary-
ing degrees of success as an alternative means of product stabilization. Penicillins are rather unstable in

aqueous solution due to β-lactam ring hydrolysis to the
corresponding penicilloic acid. Under acidic conditions the hyperallergenic, penicillenic acid can also
be formed. Injectable and oral suspension forms of
Penicillin G (CLXXXVIII) were limited due to this instability. Penicillin G degradation occurs in solution. If a sparingly soluble salt of the penicillin is
employed, then the degradation becomes zero order,
since the concentration of penicillin in the solution
remains small and constant due to replenishment of the
degraded penicillin from the suspension. Therefore,
the rate of degradation is a function of the amount of
dissolved penicillin which, in turn, is a function of
the solubility product of the salt. The benzathine,
procaine, and hydrabamine salts of various penicillins
(CLXXXIX, XCC and XCCI respectively) have been used as
sparingly soluble salts of penicillins for both oral
and I.M. administration (7-11). For Penicillin G
CLXXXIX has an aqueous solubility of 0.15 mg/ml, XCC
0.4 mg/ml, XCCI 0.075 mg/ml. These sparingly water
soluble penicillin salts which allowed the preparation
of liquid penicillin dosage forms also led to more sustained or prolonged release forms of penicillin useful
as single dose I.M. injection (7).

As stated earlier, propoxyphene (XCCII) was unstable in aqueous solution so preventing its use in a pediatric liquid dosage form. The napsylate salt of propoxyphene (Darvon-N®, XCCIII) as a sparingly soluble
salt of XCCII was formulated in a pediatric suspension
(508). XCCIII showed release characteristics of
XCCII from the suspension and capsule dosage forms
very similar to the previously used XCCII hydrochloride. However, there did appear to be a slight and expected prolonged release effect.

Erythromycin is degraded very rapidly under acidic
conditions (166). Nelson has shown that the bioavailability of erythromycin from various erythromycin esters is inversely proportional to the aqueous solubility of the esters. That is, the less water soluble the
ester, the better the bioavailability (166).

The three examples just given represent one mode
of product stabilization via the pro-drug approach.
Stabilization of a product through covalent chemical
modification by blocking a decomposition site or blocking a functional group which facilitates the decomposition has also been tried. Hetacillin, a more stable
pro-drug form of ampicillin, will be discussed later by
Dr. Sinkula. Epinephrine (IX), the catecholamine discussed earlier, is susceptible to pH dependent oxidation (518). Attempted stabilization of IX by the addi-

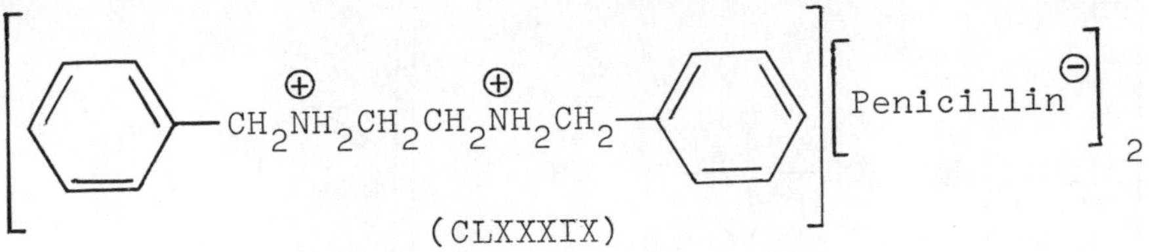

$$\left[\bigcirc\!\!-CH_2\overset{\oplus}{N}H_2CH_2CH_2\overset{\oplus}{N}H_2CH_2-\bigcirc \right]\left[\text{Penicillin}^\ominus \right]_2$$

(CLXXXIX)

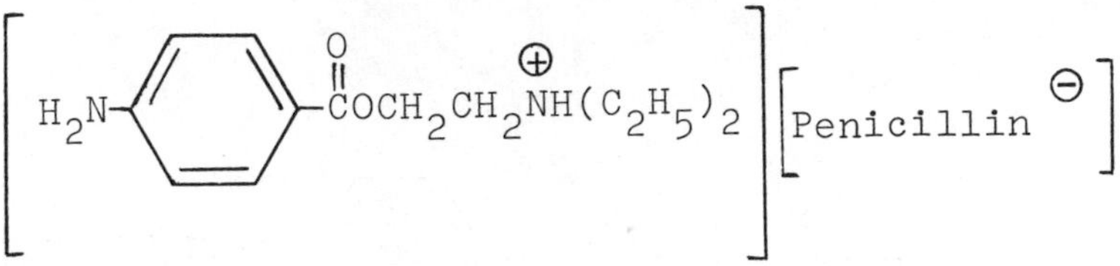

$$\left[H_2N-\bigcirc\!\!-\overset{O}{\overset{\parallel}{C}}OCH_2CH_2\overset{\oplus}{N}H(C_2H_5)_2 \right]\left[\text{Penicillin}^\ominus \right]$$

(XCC)

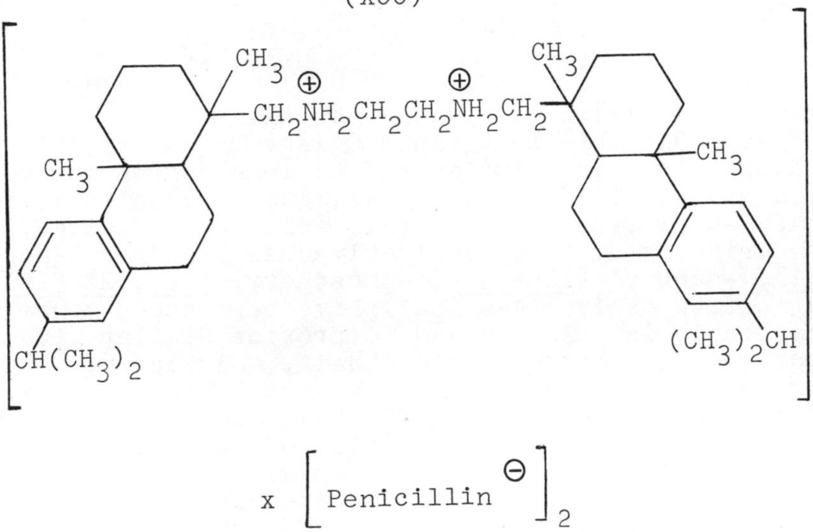

$$x\left[\text{Penicillin}^\ominus \right]_2$$

(XCCI)

tion of the antioxidant, sodium bisulfite, was found to catalyze a nonoxidative breakdown of IX to a sulfonate (XCCIV). This catalysis was studied by Higuchi and Schroeter (519) who found that the p-hydroxy group of IX was necessary for the sulfonation reaction to occur. Riegelman and Fischer (520) found that the addition of boric acid buffer to a solution of IX stabilized IX against bisulfite attack. They postulated and later isolated epinephryl borate (XCCV), a stabi-

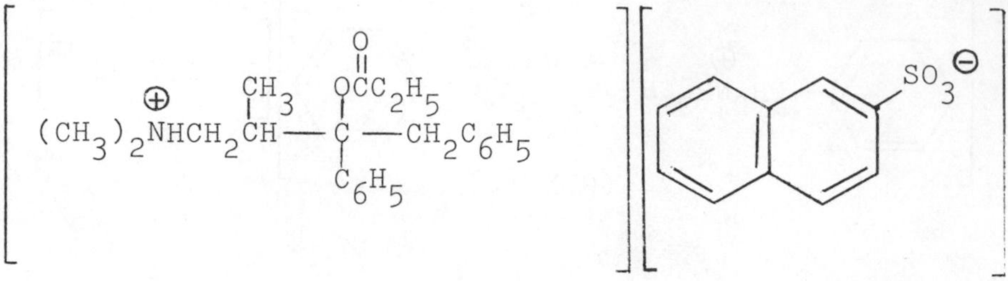

(XCCIII)

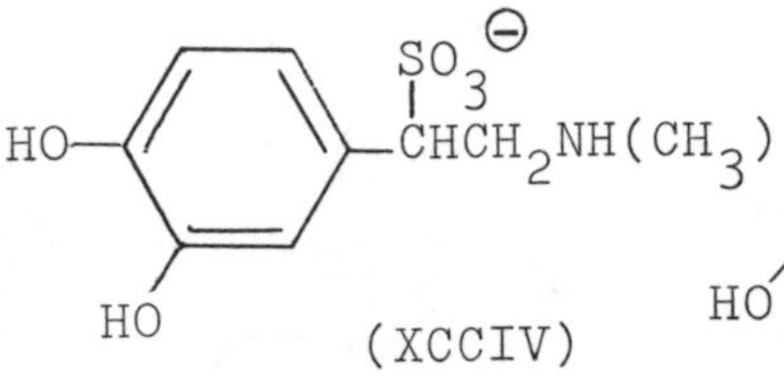

(XCCIV) 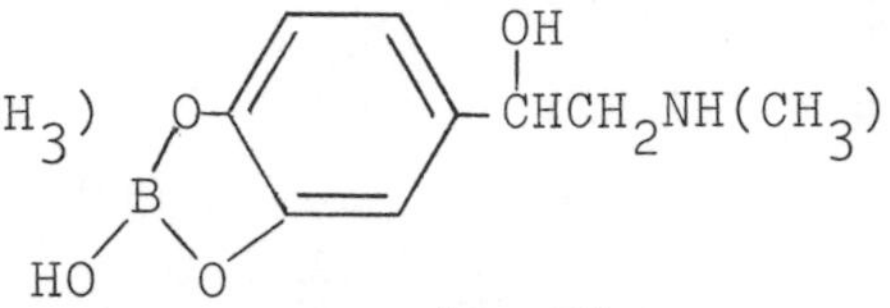   (XCCV)

lized bioreversible derivative of IX.

Ascorbic acid or vitamin C is very susceptible to
oxidation both in solution and to some degree in the
solid state. This oxidation will take place only if
the 2,3-diol system of ascorbic acid is free, i.e.,
not derivatized. Such derivatives as 2 and/or 3-acyl
(521), -benzoyl (129-132), -phosphoryl (189,522-524),
and sulfate derivatives (525) have been shown to be
more stable in solution and to provide similar vitamin
C activity as ascorbic acid itself. Similarly, various
bioreversible derivatives of hydrocortisone have been
shown to be quite stable (382-384), whereas hydrocortisone itself is quite susceptible to degradation (526).

Solid state degradations can also be a problem
with some drugs. Highly unsaturated hydrocarbons, such
as vitamin A and vitamin D, are susceptible to degradation. Guillory and Higuchi (527) studied the solid
state stability of some vitamin A derivatives. They
found that the solid state stability was inversely proportional to the melting point of the solid, i.e., the
higher the melting point of the derivative the more
stable the product. However, as stated by the authors,
the higher melting point derivatives also had the lower
aqueous solubility so the bioavailability of the more
stable products might present some problems.

Forlano et al. (528-530) studied the effect of
acylation of vitamin A alcohol on the stability of
vitamin A. The α,α-dimethylpalmityl derivative was
found to be quite stable. The biological availability

of vitamin A from the sterically hindered esters using cod liver oil and vitamin A palmitate as controls, was lower than the controls. The highest activity resulted from vitamin A palmitate with the α,α-dimethylpalmitate derivative giving 70% biological activity relative to the palmitate derivative (530).

Thiamine, or vitamin B_1, was found to be unstable when added to polished rice. Higuchi and Windheuser (92) have shown thiamine to be a very unstable compound. Various lipid soluble, stable thiamine prodrugs, such as XX-XXIV, have been found useful as food additives (91-93).

The physical and chemical properties of a drug may prevent its formulation. For example, the drug ethyl mercaptan (C_2H_5-SH, XCCVI), was found to be useful in the treatment of tuberculosis and leprosy (531). However, XCCVI has a very low boiling point of 35° which creates obvious formulation problems. Similarly, because of its odor and high vapor pressure, a problem of patient acceptance was created. Davies et al. (532-533) overcame the problem by preparing a series of thioesters, the most favorable being diethyldithiolisophthalate (XCCVII). XCCVII was a high boiling, relative-

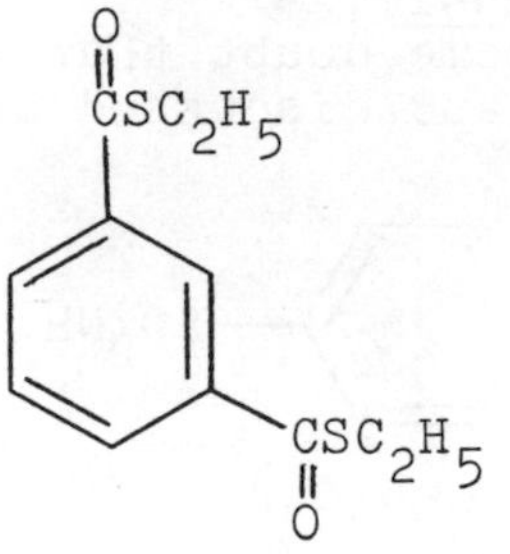

(XCCVII)

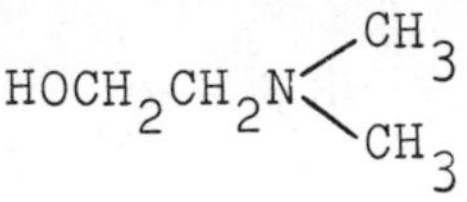

(XCCVIII)

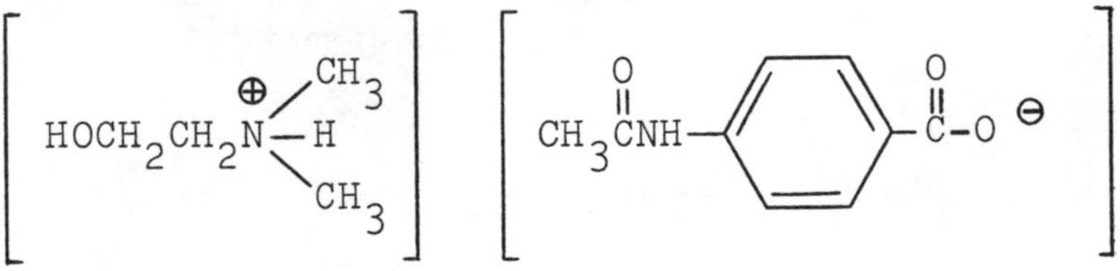

(XCCIX)

ly odorless liquid, which was administered by enunction and on absorption reverted to XCCVI and isophthalic acid. Similarly the liquid trichloroethanol was formulated as either CLXXVIII (500), CLXXXI (501), CLXXXII (502) or CLXXIII (497-498). Another low boiling point liquid N,N-dimethylaminoethanol or deanol (XCCVIII) was formulated as its acetamidobenzoate salt (XCCIX, 534). The formulation of formaldehyde as I, CXXX, and CXXXI has already been discussed.

"Accidental" Pro-Drugs

Many of the examples that have been discussed in this paper did not result from a planned approach to the optimizing of drug delivery but were the result of accidents. Prontosil (CC), the compound that provided the clue that led to the development of sulfanilamide (CCI) and subsequently sulfonamide antimicrobial agents, was not a preconceived pro-drug of sulfanilamide (535). Similarly, it was not initially realized that oxazepam (CLVII) was a metabolite of diazepam (405-408), that phenacetin gave rise to acetaminophen (CLXXVI) (536-538), that phenylbutazone had an active metabolite oxyphenbutazone (539), and that zoxazolamine was metabolized to chlorzoxazone which also possessed muscle relaxant properties (540-541).

At the same time there is some doubt that some of the examples generally accepted and discussed as pro-

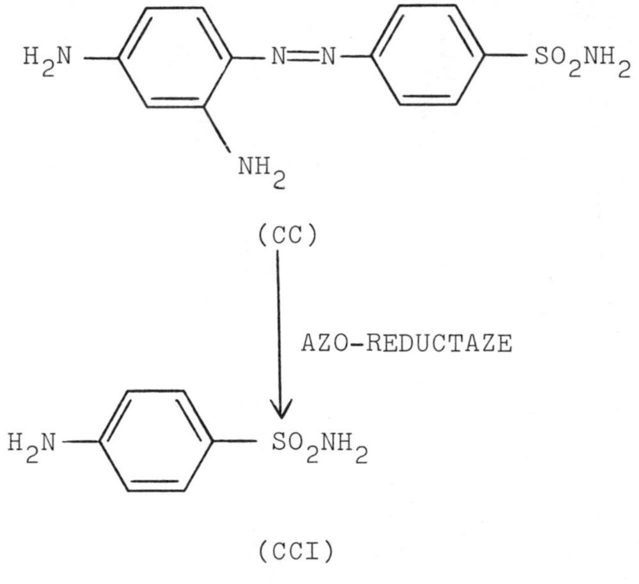

$$H_2N - \langle ring \rangle - N=N - \langle ring \rangle - SO_2NH_2$$

with NH_2 substituent

(CC)

AZO-REDUCTAZE

$$H_2N - \langle ring \rangle - SO_2NH_2$$

(CCI)

drugs are truly pro-drugs. The carbamates of mephen-
isn and the 2-substituted propanediols may have muscle
relaxant and anticonvulsant activity of their own (542,
543). For example, there is no proof that adriamycin-
14-octanoate (CLXV) exerts its cytoxic activity due to
conversion to adriamycin (429). To prove that a derivative exerts its activity as a result of conversion to
the parent compound or some other metabolite is not an
easy task.

Conclusion

     As has been demonstrated in this review, the pro-
drug concept has produced many useful and potentially
useful drugs. It must be remembered that in making any
chemical modification we are still dependent on the
mode of administration of the drug. Fluphenazine decanoate is only useful as a long acting antipsychotic
drug if given as an I.M. injection in an oil vehicle
(318). The solving of one problem may create another.
The dextran iron complex with all its advantages over
ionic iron was at one stage suspected of causing sar-
comas (544). Solving one problem via a technique can
lead to other benefits. Benzathine penicillin, which
provided a liquid dosage form of penicillin, also led
to a more sustained or prolonged release form of penicillin on I.M. injection (7).
     As the FDA in the USA and governing agencies in
other countries become more stringent with new drug applications, many companies are turning to the pro-drug
approach to both improve the efficiency and safety of
delivery of new products and to help gain further patent coverage on older products which had shown deficiencies. Whether new drug applications for pro-drugs
of some older, well established products will be easier
to obtain is uncertain.
     A problem that is now well recognized is that many
useful drugs have been rejected because, in the screening process, less than the ideal dosage form for the
drug was used. A rather active drug may have been
overlooked simply because its poor aqueous solubility
did not allow a sufficient amount of the drug to be absorbed. Of course, it would be an arduous and impractical task to make pro-drugs of each and every entity
as it appears. However, if an agent is suspected to be
highly active based on some structure-activity rela-
tionship (SAR) or preliminary testing, but suffers from
poor solubility or some other limitation, the possible
development of pro-drugs at an early stage may provide
for greater success in the screening of active medici-

nal agents.

All the implications just discussed make the area of pro-drugs an exciting and fruitful field for continued study. It is an area where the pharmaceutical chemist, with his knowledge and expertise in solubility theory, pharmacokinetics and formulation variables, the medicinal chemist, with his knowledge of synthesis, SAR and metabolism, and the pharmacologist, with his knowledge of mechanisms and sites of drug action and toxicity can cooperate to optimize the delivery of an active drug to its site of action while minimizing toxicity and unfavorable reactions to the drug. Many problems associated with drugs can be overcome by the use of pro-drug approach, and it is the hope of this author that this review will stimulate further research in this area.

Literature Cited

1. Albert, A., Nature (1958), 182, 421.
2. Albert, A., "Selective Toxicity", pp 57-63, John Wiley and Sons Inc., New York, N.Y., 1964.
3. Harper, N. J., J. Med. Pharm. Chem. (1959), 1, 467.
4. Harper, N. J., Progr. Drug Res., (1962), 4, 221.
5. Kupchan, S. M., Casy, A. F., and Swintosky, J. V., J. Pharm. Sci. (1965), 54, 514.
6. Sinkula, A. A., and Yalkowsky, S. H., "Rationale for the Design of Biologically Reversible Drug Derivatives-Prodrugs" to be published as a review in J. Pharm. Sci., 1975.
7. Sullivan, N. P., Symmes, A. T., Miller, H. C., and Rhodehamel, Jr., H. W., Science (1948), 107, 169.
8. Hobby, G. L., Brown, E. and Patelski, R. A., Proc. Soc. Exp. Biol. Med. (1948), 67, 6.
9. Szabo, J. L., Edwards, C. D., and Bruce, W. F., Antibiot. Chemother. (1951), 1, 499.
10. Samuel, M., Science (1947), 106, 370.
11. Swintosky, J. V., Rosen, E., Robinson, M. J., Chamberlain, R. E., and Guarini, J. R., J. Amer. Pharm. Ass. Sci. Ed. (1956), 45, 37.
12. White, M. G., and Asch, M. J., N. Engl. J. Med. (1971), 284, 1281.
13. Pruit, Jr., B. A., Mancrief, J. A., and Mason, A. D., U. S. Army Institute of Surgical Research, (1967), Section 2, 1.
14. Beyer, K. H., and Gourier, G. W., Science (1945), 101, 150.
15. Ariens, E. J., Progr. Drug Res. (1966), 10, 429.
16. Ariens, E. J., Il Farmaco Ed. Sci. (1969), 24, 3.

17. Ariens, E. J., "Drug Design", Vol II, p. 2, Academic Press, New York, N. Y., 1971.

18. Ariens, E. J., "A Molecular Approach to the Modulation of Pharmacokinetics", published as a paper in "The Physiological Equivalence of Drug Dosage Forms", p. 23, presented by the Food and Drug Directorate in Ottawa, Canada, 1969.

19. Bungaard, H., Dansk Tidsskrift Farm. (1971), $\underline{45}$, 73.

20. Sinkula, A. A., "Molecular Modification: Derivative Formation and Pharmaceutical Properties", 14th Annual National Industrial Pharmaceutical Research Conference, Land O'Lakes, Wis., June, 1972.

21. Stella, V. J., Aust. J. Pharm. Sci. (1973), $\underline{NS2}$, 57.

22. Notari, R. E., J. Pharm. Sci. (1973), $\underline{62}$, 865.

23. Teorell, T., Dedrick, R. L., and Condliffe, P. G., "Pharmacology and Pharmacokinetics", Plenum Press, New York, N. Y., 1974.

24. Perrier, D., and Gibaldi, M., J. Clin. Pharmacol. (1974), $\underline{14}$, 415.

25. Gibaldi, M., Levy, G., and Weintraub, H., Clin. Pharmacol. Ther. (1971), $\underline{12}$, 734.

26. Higuchi, T., and Davis, S. S., J. Pharm. Sci. (1970), $\underline{59}$, 1376.

27. Hansch, C., "Quantitative Approaches to Pharmacological Structure-Activity Relationships", Chapt. 3, Cavallito, C. J., ed., Pergamon Press, New York, N. Y., 1973.

28. Flynn, G., Yalkowsky, S. H., and Roseman, T. J., J. Pharm. Sci. (1974), $\underline{63}$, 479.

29. Ariens, E. J., and Simonis, A. M., "Drug Action: Target Tissue, Dose-Response Relationships, and Receptors", in "Pharmacology and Pharmacokinetics" p. 163, Teorell, T., Dedrick, R. L., and Condliffe, P. G., eds., Plenum Press, New York, N. Y., 1974.

30. Perrier, D., and Gibaldi, M., J. Clin. Pharmacol. (1972), $\underline{12}$, 449.

31. Rowland, M., "Effect of Some Physiologic Factors in Bioavailability of Oral Dosage Forms," in "Dosage Form Design and Bioavailability," Chapter 6, Swarbrick, J., ed., Lea and Febiger, Philadelphia, Penn., 1973.

32. Barr, W. H., Drug Inf. Bull. (1969), 27.

33. Riegelman, S., and Sadee, W., "Which Drugs Can and Should be Monitored Today and Tomorrow" in "Clinical Pharmacokinetics", p. 169, Levy, G., ed., American Pharmaceutical Association, Washington, D. C., 1974.

34. Dollery, C. T., Davies, D. S., and Connolly, M.
    E., Ann. N. Y. Acad. Sci. (1971), 179, 108.
35. Hornykiewicz, O., Pharmacol. Rev. (1966), 18, 925.
36. Hornykiewicz, O., Pharmako-Psychiat. Neuro-Psycho-
    pharmakol. (1968), 1, 6.
37. Barbeau, A., Rev. Can. Biol. (1967), 26, 55.
38. Ernst, A. M., Acta Physiol. Pharmacol. Neerl.
    (1965), 15, 141.
39. Friedman, A. H., and Everett, G. M., Adv. Pharma-
    col. (1964), 3, 83.
40. Curzon, G., Int. Rev. Neurobiol. (1968), 10, 323.
41. Cotzias, G. C., Papavasilious, P. S., Gellene, R.,
    and Aronson, R. B., Trans. Ass. Amer. Phys. (1968)
    81, 171.
42. Cotzias, G. C., Papavasilious, P. S., and Gellene,
    R., N. Engl. J. Med. (1966), 780, 337.
43. Godwin-Austen, R. B., Tomlinson, E. B., Frears,
    C. C., and Kok, H. W. L., Lancet (1969), 2, 165.
44. Peaston, M. J., and Bianchine, J. R., Brit. Med.
    J. (1970), 1, 400.
45. Klawans, H. L., and Garvin, J. S., Dis. Nerv.
    Syst. (1969), 30, 737.
46. McDowell, F., Lee, J. E., Swift, T., Sweet, T.,
    Ogsbury, J. S., and Kessler, J. T., Ann. Intern.
    Med. (1970), 72, 29.
47. Yahr, M. D., Duvoisin, R. C., Schear, M. J.,
    Barrett, R. B., and Hoehn, M. M., Arch. Neurol.
    (1969), 21, 343.
48. Barbeau, A., Can. Med. Ass. J. (1969), 101, 91.
49. Calne, D. B., Karoum, F., Ruthven, C. R. J., and
    Sandler, M., Brit. J. Pharmacol. (1969), 37, 57.
50. Mawdsley, C., Brit. Med. J. (1970), 1, 331.
51. Yoshida, H., Namba, J., Kaniike, K., and Imaizumi,
    R., Jap. J. Pharmacol. (1963), 13, 1.
52. Shindo, H., Ann. Sankyo Res. Lab. (1972), 24, 1.
53. Kaplan, S. A., and Cotler, S., Paper 25 presented
    at the 17th National Meeting of the Academy of
    Pharmaceutical Sciences, New Orleans, 1974.
54. Bianchine, J. R., Calimlim, L. R., Morgan, J. P.,
    Dujuvne, C. A., and Lassagna, L., Ann. N. Y. Acad.
    Sci. (1971), 179, 126.
55. Imai, K., Suguira, M., Tamura, Z., Hirayama, K.,
    and Narabayshi, H., Chem. Pharm. Bull. (1971), 17,
    439.
56. Rivera-Calimlim, L., Duyuvne, C. A., Morgan, J.
    P., Lassagna, L., and Bianchine, J. R., Brit. Med.
    J. (1970), 4, 93.
57. Shindo, H., Miyakoshi, N., and Takahashi, I.,
    Chem. Pharm. Bull. (1971), 19, 2490.

58. Shindo, H., Miyakoshi, N., and Nakajima, E., Chem.
     Pharm. Bull. (1972), 20, 966.
59. Shindo, H., Komai, T., Tanaka, K., Nakajima, E.,
     and Miyakoshi, N., Chem. Pharm. Bull (1973), 21,
     826.
60. Shindo, H., Nakajima, E., Kawai, K., Miyakoshi,
     N., and Tanaka, K., Chem. Pharm. Bull. (1973), 21,
     817.
61. Lai, C. M., and Mason, W. D., J. Pharm. Sci.
     (1973), 62, 510.
62. Martin, R. B., J. Phys. Chem. (1971), 75, 2657.
63. Niebergall, P. J., Schnaare, R. L., and Sugita, E.
     T., J. Pharm. Sci. (1972), 61, 232.
64. Fung, H. L., and Cheng, L., J. Chem. Ed. (1974),
     51, 106.
65. Riegelman, S., Strait, L. A., and Fischer, E. Z.,
     J. Pharm. Sci. (1962), 51, 129.
66. Edsall, J. T., Martin, R. B., and Hollingworth, B.
     R., Proc. Nat. Acad. Sci. (1958), 44, 505.
67. Andén, N. E., Corrodi, D. L., Dahlström, A., Fuxe,
     K., and Hökfelt, T., Life Sciences (1966), 5, 561.
68. Pinder, R. M., Nature (1970), 228, 358.
69. Creveling, C. R., Daly, J. W., Tokuyama, T., and
     Witkop, B., Experientia (1969), 25, 26.
70. Daly, J. W., Creveling, C. R., and Witkop, B., J.
     Med. Chem. (1966), 9, 273.
71. Borgman, R. J., McPhillips, J. J., Stitzel, R. E.,
     and Goodman, I. J., J. Med. Chem. (1973), 16, 630.
72. Goldberg, L. I., Talley, R. C., McNay, J. L.,
     Progr. Cardiovasc. Dis. (1969), 12, 40.
73. Marchetti, G., Merlo, L., Noseda, V., G. Ital.
     Cardiol. (1971), 1, 49.
74. Casagrande, C., and Ferrari, G., Il Farmaco Ed.
     Sci. (1973), 28, 143.
75. Jones, P. H., Biel, J. H., Ours, C. W., Klundt, L.,
     and Lenga, R. L., Paper and abstract presented at
     the 165th meeting of the Amer. Chem. Soc., MEDI 9,
     (1973).
76. Verbiscar, A. J., and Abood, L. G., J. Med. Chem.
     (1970), 13, 1176.
77. Bjurlf, P., Carlström, S., and Rorsman, G., Acta
     Med. Scand. (1967), 182, 273.
78. Kupchan, S. M., and Isenberg, A. C., J. Med. Chem.
     (1967), 10, 960.
79. Mayer, S., Maickel, R. P., and Brodie, B. B., J.
     Pharmacol. Exp. Ther. (1959), 127, 205.
80. Brodie, B. B., Kurz, H., and Schanker, L. S., J.
     Pharmacol. Exp. Ther. (1960), 130, 20.
81. Hansch, C., Steward, A. R., Anderson, S. M., and
     Bentley, D., J. Med. Chem. (1968), 11, 1.

82. Bertler, A., Falck, B., Owman, C., and Rosengrenn, E., Pharmacol. Rev. (1966), 18, 369.
83. Cohen, S., Vzan, A., and Valette, G., Biochem. Pharmacol. (1962), 11, 721.
84. Rindi, G., and Ventura, U., Physiol. Rev. (1972), 52, 821.
85. Thomson, A. D., Baker, H., and Leevy, C. M., J. Lab. Clin. Med. (1970), 76, 34.
86. Thomson, A. D., Baker, H., and Leevy, C. M., Amer. J. Clin. Nutr. (1968), 21, 537.
87. Tomasulo, P. A., and Kater, R. M. H., Amer. J. Clin. Nutr. (1968), 21, 1341.
88. Thomson, A. D., Frank, O., Baker, H., and Leevy, C. M., Ann. Intern. Med. (1971), 74, 529.
89. Pincus, J. H., Develop. Med. Child Neurol. (1972), 14, 87.
90. Montpetit, V. J. A., Anderman, F., Carpenter, S., Fawcett, J. S., Zborowska-slvis, D., and Giverson, H. R., Brain (1971), 94, 1.
91. Matsukawa, T., Yurugi, S., and Oka, Y., Ann. N. Y. Acad. Sci. (1962), 92, 430.
92. Windheuser, J. J., and Higuchi, T., J. Pharm. Sci. (1962), 51, 354.
93. Kawasaki, C., Vitam. Horm. (1963), 21, 69.
94. Nogami, H., Hasegawa, J., and Riheshisa, T., Chem. Pharm. Bull. (1973), 21, 858.
95. Nogami, H., Hasegawa, J., and Noda, K., Chem. Pharm. Bull. (1969), 17, 219.
96. Nogami, H., Hasegawa, J., and Noda, K., Chem. Pharm. Bull. (1969), 17, 228.
97. Nogami, H., Hasegawa, J., and Noda, K., Chem. Pharm. Bull. (1969), 17, 234.
98. Grode, G. A., Falb, R. D., Crowley, J. P., and Truitt, E. B., Pharmacol. (1974), 11, 102.
99. Iwasaki, T., Vitamins (Kyoto) (1955), 9, 525.
100. Stella, V., Unpublished results.
101. Matsubara, K., Vitamins (Kyoto) (1957), 12, 80.
102. Takenouchi, K., Aso, K., Shimizu, S., and Kobayashi, T., Vitamins (Kyoto) (1962), 26, 245.
103. Takenouchi, K., Aso, K., Shimizu, S., and Kobayashi, T., Vitamins (Kyoto) (1962), 26, 251.
104. Takenouchi, K., Aso, K., Shimizu, S., and Kobayashi, T., Vitamins (Kyoto) (1962), 26, 257.
105. Takenouchi, K., Aso, K., Shimizu, S., and Kobayashi, T., Vitamins (Kyoto) (1962), 26, 261.
106. Takenouchi, K., Aso, K., and Nazaki, Y., Vitamins (Kyoto) (1962), 26, 222.
107. Takenouchi, K., Aso, K., Minato, A., and Hirose, S., Vitamins (Kyoto) (1962), 26, 241.

108. Morita, M., and Minesita, T., Vitamins (Kyoto) (1966), 33, 61.
109. Takamizawa, A., and Harai, K., Chem. Pharm. Bull. (1962), 10, 1102.
110. Takamizawa, A., Inazu, K., Nakanishi, S., Ito, H., Sato, H., Ando, M., Akahori, A., and Yamamoto, R., Ann. Rept. Shionogi Res. Lab. (1967), 17, 59.
111. Minesita, T., Morita, M., and Iwata, T., Vitamins (Kyoto) (1962), 25, 483.
112. Miyagawa, K., Mujamoto, T., and Murata, K., Vitamins (Kyoto) (1962), 26, 31.
113. Suzuoki, Z., Suzuoki, T., and Kurihara, M., Vitamins (Kyoto) (1962), 7, 118.
114. Howard, L., Wagner, C., and Schenker, S., J. Nutr. (1974), 104, 1024.
115. Levy, A., and Hewitt, R. R., Amer. J. Clin. Nutr. (1971), 24, 401.
116. Chang, T., Lewis, J., and Glazko, A. J., Biochim. Biophys. Acta (1967), 135, 1000.
117. Israel, Y., Salazar, I., and Rosenmann, E., J. Nutr. (1968), 96, 499.
118. Israel, Y., Valenzuela, J. E., Salazar, I., and Vgarte, G., J. Nutr. (1970), 98, 222.
119. Yagi, K., Okuda, J., Dmitrovskii, A. A., Honda, R., and Matsubara, T., J. Vitaminol. (1961), 7, 276.
120. Yagi, K., Yamamoto, Y., and Okuda, J., Nature (1961), 191, 171.
121. Shintani, S., Tanaka, F., Nakamura, M., and Sato, M, J. Vitaminol. (1961), 7, 182.
122. Shintani, S., Tanaka, F., Nakamura, M., and Sato, M., J. Vitaminol. (1961), 7, 122.
123. Editorial, Jap. Med. Gaz. (1965), 2, 12.
124. Isler, O., Experientia (1970), 26, 225.
125. Swern, D., Stirton, A. J., and Wells, P. A., Oil and Soap (1943), 20, 224.
126. Kulesza, J., Gora, J., and Drygier, J., Zesz. Nachem. Spozyw. (1967), 12, 29. Through Chem. Abst. (1967), 67, 117165g.
127. Misaka, S., Tsuji, N., Seo, S., and Iijima, S., Tokyo Ikadaiguku-zasshi (1960), 18, 1743.
128. Feldheim, W., and Czerny, M., Biochem. Z. (1959), 331, 150.
129. Imai, Y., Chem. Pharm. Bull. (1966), 14, 1045.
130. Imai, Y., Matsumura, H., and Aramaki, Y., Jap. J. Pharmacol. (1967), 17, 330.
131. Nomura, H., and Sugimoto, K., Chem. Pharm. Bull. (1966), 14, 1039.
132. Hoffman-LaRoche and Co., Ger. Pat. 701561 (1940).

133. Bloch, A., "The Design of Biologically Active
      Nucleosides"in "Drug Design", Vol. IV, Chapt. 8,
      Ariens, E. J., ed., Academic Press, New York, N.
      Y., 1973.
134. Welch, A. D., Cancer Res. (1961), 21, 1475.
135. Sorm, F., Beranek, J., Smrt, J., Krupicka, J.,
      and Skoda, J., Collection Czech. Chem. Commun.
      (1962), 27, 575.
136. Chladek, S., Sorm, F., and Smrt, J., Collection
      Czech. Chem. Commun. (1962), 27, 87.
137. Zemlicka, J., Beranek, J., and Smrt, J., Collec-
      tion Czech. Chem. Commun. (1962), 27, 2784.
138. Beranek, J., and Pitha, J., Collection Czech.
      Chem. Commun. (1964), 29, 625.
139. Ceskoslovenska Akademic Ved (by Beranek, J., and
      Sorm, F.), Belgian Pat., 639,341 (1964).
140. Grafnettorova, J., Beranek, J., Koenig, J.,
      Smahel, O., and Sorm, F., Neoplasma (1966), 13,
      241.
141. Turner, R. W., and Calabresi, P., J. Invest. Der-
      matol. (1964), 43, 551.
142. Saksena, S. K., and Chaudhury, R. R., Indian J.
      Med. Res. (1969), 57, 1940.
143. Hoeksema, H., Whitfield, G. B., and Rhuland, L.
      E., Biochem. Biophys. Res. Commun. (1961), 6,
      213.
144. Posternak, T., Sutherland, E. W., and Henion, W.
      F., Biochim. Biophys. Acta (1962), 65, 558.
145. Haskell, T. H., and Hanessian, S., U. S. Patent
      3,651,045 (1972).
146. Gerzon, K., and Kau, D., J. Med. Chem. (1967),
      10, 189.
147. Levine, R. R., and Pelkin, E. W., J. Pharmacol.
      Exp. Ther. (1961), 131, 319.
148. Levine, R. R., J. Pharmacol. Exp. Ther. (1960),
      129, 296.
149. Levine, R. R., Weinstock, J., Zirckle, C. S., and
      McClean, R., J. Pharmacol. Exp. Ther. (1961),
      131, 334.
150. Streitwieser, Jr., A., Chem. Rev. (1950), 56,
      667.
151. Kusnetsov, S. G., and Ioffe, D. B., J. Gen. Chem.
      USSR (1961), 31, 2289.
152. Ross, S. B., and Fröden, Ö., Europ. J. Pharmacol.
      (1970), 13, 46.
153. Ross, S. B., Johansson, J. G., Lindborg, B., and
      Dahlbom, R., Acta Pharm. Suecica (1973), 10, 29.
154. Johansson, J. G., Lindborg, B., Dahlbom, R.,
      Ross, S. B., and Akerman, B. A., Acta Pharm.
      Suecica (1973), 10, 199.

155. Ross, S. B., Sandberg, R., Akerman, B. A., Domeii, K. E., Stening, G., and Suensson, S., J. Med. Chem. (1973), 16, 787.

156. Lindborg, B., Johansson, J. G., Dahlbom, R., and Ross, S. B., Acta Pharm. Suecica (1974), 11, 401.

157. Ross, S. B., and Akerman, S. B. A., J. Pharmacol. Exp. Ther. (1972), 182, 351.

158. Kirby, W. M. M., and Kind, C., Ann. N. Y. Acad. Sci. (1967), 145, 291.

159. Kunin, C. M., Ann. N. Y. Acad. Sci. (1967), 145, 282.

160. Daehne, W. V., Frederiksen, E., Gundersen, E., Lund, F., Mørch, P., Petersen, H. J., Roholt, K., Tybring, L., and Godtfredsen, W. O., J. Med. Chem. (1970), 13, 607.

161. Klein, J. O., and Finland, M., Amer. J. Med. Sci. (1963), 66, 544.

162. Modr, Z., and Dvoracek, K., Rev. Czech. Med. (1970), 16, 84.

163. Loo, J. C. K., Foltz, E. L., Wallick, H., and Kwan, K. C., Clin. Pharmacol. Ther. (1974), 16, 35.

164. Perrier, D., and Gibaldi, M., J. Pharm. Sci. (1973), 62, 1486.

165. Chun, A. H. C., and Seitz, J. A., J. Amer. Pharm. Ass. (1974), NS14, 407.

166. Nelson, E., Chem. Pharm. Bull. (1962), 10, 1099.

167. Smith, J. W., Dyke, R. W., and Griffith, R. S., J. Amer. Med. Ass. (1953), 151, 805.

168. Shubin, H., Dumas, K., and Sokmensuer, A., Antibiot. Ann. (1957-1958), 679.

169. Meyer, C. E., and Lewis, C., "Antimicrobial Agents and Chemotherapy", American Society for Microbiology (1963), 169.

170. Wagner, J. G., Can. J. Pharm. Sci. (1966), 1, 55.

171. Sobin, B. A., English, A. R., and Celmer, W. D., Antibiot. Ann. (1954-1955), 827.

172. Celmer, W. D., Els, H., and Murray, K., Antibiot. Ann. (1957-1958), 476.

173. Celmer, W. D., Antibiot. Ann. (1958-1959), 277.

174. English, A. R., and McBride, T. J., Antibiot. Chemother. (1958), 8, 424.

175. English, A. R., and McBride, T. J., Proc. Soc. Exp. Biol. Med. (1959), 100, 880.

176. Smith, I. M., and Soderstrom, W. H., J. Amer. Med. Ass. (1959), 170, 184.

177. Stephens, V. C., Antibiot. Ann. (1953-1954), 514.

178. Murphy, H. W., Antibiot. Ann. (1953-1954), 500.

179. Clark, R. K., and Varner, E. L., Antibiot. Chemother. (1957), 7, 487.

180. Jones, P. H., Perun, T. J., Rowley, E. K., and
     Baker, E. J., J. Med. Chem. (1972), 15, 631.
181. Martin, Y. C., Jones, P. H., Perun, T. J.,
     Grundy, W. E., Bell, S., Bower, R. R., and Ship-
     kowitz, N. L., J. Med. Chem. (1972), 15, 635.
182. Tardew, P. L., Mao, J. C. H., and Kennedy, D.,
     Appl. Microbiol. (1969), 18, 159.
183. Fletcher, H. P., Murray, H. M., and Weddon, T.
     E., J. Pharm. Sci. (1968), 57, 2101.
184. Morozowich, W., Sinkula, A. A., MacKellar, F. A.,
     and Lewis, C., J. Pharm. Sci. (1973), 62, 1102.
185. Sinkula, A. A., and Lewis, C., J. Pharm. Sci.
     (1973), 62, 1757.
186. Málek, P., Kolc, J., Herold, M., and Hoffman, J.,
     Antibiot. Ann. (1957-1958), 546.
187. Foreman, H., "Metal Binding in Medicine", p. 82,
     Seven, M. J., ed., Lippincott, Philadelphia,
     Penn., 1960.
188. Catsch, A., Fed. Proc. (1961), 20, part II, 206.
189. Imai, Y., Usui, T., Matsuzaki, T., Yokotani, H.,
     Mima, H., and Aramaki, Y., Jap. J. Pharmacol.
     (1967), 17, 317.
190. "American Hospital Formulary Service", American
     Society Hospital Pharmacists, Washington, D. C.
     (1974), 84, 04.16.
191. Perrin, D. D., "Dissociation Constants of Organic
     Bases in Aqueous Solution", p. 119, Butterworth
     Co., London, England, 1965.
192. Barry, B. W., and Woodford, R., Brit. J. Derma-
     tol. (1974), 91, 323.
193. "American Hospital Formulary Service", American
     Society Hospital Pharmacists, Washington, D. C.
     (1974), 84, 06.
194. Poulsen, B., "Design of Topical Drug Products:
     Biopharmaceutics", in "Drug Design", Vol. IV,
     Chapt. 5, Ariens, E. J., ed., Academic Press,
     New York, N. Y., 1973.
195. Maistrello, I., Rigamonti, G., Frova, C., and de
     Ruggieri, P., J. Pharm. Sci. (1973), 62, 1455.
196. Fed. Regist. (1974), 39, 2471.
197. Wagner, J. G., Christensen, M., Sakmar, E., Blair,
     D., Yates, J. D., Willis, III, P. W., Sedman, A.
     J., and Stoll, R. G., J. Amer. Med. Ass. (1973),
     224, 199.
198. Skelly, J., and Knapp, G., J. Amer. Med. Ass.
     (1973), 224, 243.
199. Lindenbaum, J., Mellow, M. G., Blackstone, M. D.,
     and Butler, P., N. Engl. J. Med. (1971), 285,
     1344.

200. Vitti, T. G., Banes, D., and Byers, T. E., N.
     Engl. J. Med. (1971), <u>285</u>, 1433.
201. Higuchi, T., and Ikeda, M., J. Pharm. Sci. (1974),
     <u>63</u>, 809.
202. Noyes, A. A., and Whitney, W. R., J. Amer. Chem.
     Soc. (1897), <u>19</u>, 930.
203. Rietbrock, N., Abshagen, U., Bergmann, K. V., and
     Kewitz, H., Naunyn Schmiedebergs Arch. Pharmacol.
     (1972), <u>274</u>, 171.
204. Rietbrock, N., Rennekamp, C., Rennekamp, H.,
     Bergmann, K. V., and Abshagen, U., Naunyn
     Schmiedebergs Arch. Pharmacol. (1972), <u>272</u>, 450.
205. Rennekamp, H., Rennekamp, C., Abshagen, U.,
     Bergmann, K. V., and Rietbrock, N., Naunyn
     Schmiedebergs Arch. Pharmacol. (1972), <u>273</u>, 172.
206. Stoll, A., and Kreis, W., Schweiz. Med. Wschr.
     (1953), <u>83</u>, 266.
207. Rothlin, E., Bircher, R., and Schalch, W. R.,
     Schweiz. Med. Wschr. (1953), <u>83</u>, 267.
208. Haberland, G., Arzneim. Forsch. (1965), <u>15</u>, 481.
209. Greef, K., Schwarzmann, D., and Waschulzik, G.,
     Arzneim. Forsch. (1965), <u>15</u>, 483.
210. Benthe, H. F., Arzneim. Forsch. (1965), <u>15</u>, 486.
211. Förster, W., and Schulzeck, S., Biochem. Pharma-
     col. (1968), <u>17</u>, 489.
212. Cloetta, M., Arch. Exp. Path. Pharmak. (1926),
     <u>112</u>, 261.
213. Fiehring, H., Knappe, J., and Sundermann, A.,
     Dt. Ges. Wesen. (1964), <u>19</u>, 2439.
214. Georges, A., Pape, J., and Duvernay, G., Arch.
     Int. Pharmacodyn. Ther. (1966), <u>164</u>, 47.
215. Ishaq, K. S., and Gisvold, O., J. Pharm. Sci.
     (1970), <u>59</u>, 412.
216. Megges, S. R., and Repke, K., Naunyn Schmiede-
     bergs Arch. Exp. Path. Pharmak. (1961), <u>241</u>, 534.
217. White, W. F., and Gisvold, O., J. Amer. Pharm.
     Ass. Sci. Ed. (1952), <u>41</u>, 42.
218. Hussain, A., and Rytting, J. H., J. Pharm. Sci.
     (1974), <u>63</u>, 798.
219. Atkinson, R. M., Bedford, C., Child, K. J., and
     Tomich, E. G., Antibiot. Chemother. (1962), <u>12</u>,
     232.
220. Crounze, R. G., J. Invest. Dermatol. (1961), <u>37</u>,
     529.
221. McNall, E. G., Antibiot. Ann. (1959-1960), <u>7</u>,
     674.
222. Gonzalez-Ochoa, A., and Ahumada - Padilla, M.,
     Arch. Dermatol. (1960), <u>81</u>, 833.
223. Sharpe, H. M., and Tomich, E. G., Toxicol. Appl.
     Pharmacol. (1960), <u>2</u>, 44.

224. Bedford, C., Busfield, D., Child, K. J., Mac-
      Gregor, I., Sutherland, P., and Tomich, E. G.,
      Arch. Dermatol. (1960), 81, 735.
225. Chiou, W. L., and Riegelman, S., J. Pharm. Sci.
      (1971), 60, 1376.
226. Carrigan, P. J., and Bates, T. R., J. Pharm. Sci.
      (1973), 62, 1476.
227. Fischer, L. J., and Riegelman, S., J. Pharm. Sci.
      (1967), 56, 469.
228. Williams, R. T., "Detoxification Mechanisms", p.
      166, John Wiley and Sons, Inc., New York, N. Y.,
      1959.
229. Magee, W. E., Armour, S. B., and Miller, O. V.,
      Biochim. Biophys. Acta (1973), 306, 270.
230. Karim, S. M. M., and Sharma, S. D., J. Obstect.
      Gynaec. Commun. (1972), 79, 737.
231. Schedl, H. P., and Clifton, J. A., Gastroenterol.
      (1961), 41, 491.
232. Tanabe, M., and Bigley, B., J. Amer. Chem. Soc.
      (1961), 83, 756.
233. Fried, J., Borman, A., Kessler, W. B., Grabowich,
      P., and Sabo, E. F., J. Amer. Chem. Soc. (1958),
      80, 2338.
234. Gardi, R., Vitali, R., and Ercoli, A., J. Org.
      Chem. (1962), 27, 668.
235. Heller, U. S. Patent 3,608,076 (1971), through
      Wilbur, R. D. (to American Cyanamid Co.), U. S.
      Patent 3,772,435 (1973).
236. Anderson, E., Haymaker, W., and Henderson, E.,
      J. Amer. Med. Ass. (1940), 115, 2167.
237. Gardi, R., Vitali, R., Falconi, G., and Ercoli,
      A., J. Med. Chem. (1973), 16, 123.
238. Zaks, A., Jones, T., Fink, M., and Freedman, A.
      M., J. Amer. Med. Ass. (1971), 215, 2108.
239. Dayton, P. B., and Blumberg, H., Fed. Proc. Fed.
      Amer. Soc. Exp. Biol. (1970), 29, 686.
240. Linder, C., and Fishman, J., J. Med. Chem. (1973),
      16, 553.
241. Editorial, Chem. Eng. News (1972), 14.
242. Way, E. L., and Adler, T. K., Pharmacol. Rev.
      (1960), 12, 383.
243. Kupchan, S. M., and Casy, A. F., J. Med. Chem.
      (1967), 10, 959.
244. Yoshimura, H., Oguri, K., and Tsukamoto, H.,
      Biochem. Pharmacol. (1969), 18, 279.
245. Oguri, K., Ida, S., Yoshimura, H., and Tsukamoto,
      H., Chem. Pharm. Bull. (1970), 18, 2414.
246. Mori, M., Oguri, K., Yoshimura, H., Shimomura, K.,
      Kamata, O., and Ueki, S., Life Sciences (1972),
      11, 525.

247. Field, L., and Sweetman, B. J., J. Org. Chem. (1969), 34, 1799.

248. Field, L., Sweetman, B. J., and Bellas, M., J. Org. Chem. (1969), 12, 62.

249. Sweetman, B. J., Bellas, M., and Field, L., J. Med. Chem. (1969), 12, 888.

250. Srivastava, P. K., and Field, L., J. Med. Chem. (1973), 16, 428.

251. Hartles, R. L., and Williams, R. T., Biochem. J. (1949), 44, 335.

252. Siuda, J. F., and Cihonski, C. D., J. Pharm. Sci. (1972), 61, 1856.

253. Wagner, J. G., Holmes, T. D., Wilkinson, P. K., Blair, D. C., and Stoll, R. G., Amer. Rev. Resp. Dis. (1973), 108, 536.

254. Gibson, M. O. J., and Nagley, M. M., Tubercle (1955), 36, 209.

255. Jeker, K., Lauewer, H., Regli, J., and Friedrich, T., Amer. Rev. Tub. Pul. Dis. (1959), 79, 351.

256. Chiou, C. Y., Biochem. Pharmacol. (1971), 20, 2401.

257. Stempel, E., "Dispensing of Medication", pp. 1002-1042, Martin, E., ed., Mack Pub. Co., Easton, Penn., 1971.

258. Gray, G. D., Nichol, F. R., Mickelson, M. M., Camiener, G. W., Gish, D. T., Kelly, R. C., Wechter, W. J. Moxley, T. E., and Neil, G. L., Biochem. Pharmacol. (1972), 21, 465.

259. Warner, D. T., Neil, G. L., Taylor, A. J., and Wechter, W. J., J. Med. Chem. (1972), 15, 790.

260. Neil, G. L., Buskirk, H. H., Moxley, T. E., Manak, R. C., Kuentzel, S. L., and Bhuyan, B. K., Biochem. Pharmacol. (1971), 20, 3295.

261. Gish, D. T., Kelly, R. C., Camiener, G. W., and Wechter, W. J., J. Med. Chem. (1971), 14, 1159.

262. Neil, G. L., Wiley, P. F., Manak, R. C., and Moxley, T. E., Cancer Res. (1970), 30, 1047.

263. Tanaka, T., Kobayashi, H., Okumura, K., Muranishi, S., and Sezaki, H., Chem. Pharm. Bull. (1974), 22, 1275.

264. James, K. C., Nicholls, P. J., and Roberts, M., J. Pharm. Pharmacol. (1969), 21, 24.

265. Miescher, K., Wettstein, A., and Tschopp, E., Biochem. J. (1936), 30, 1977.

266. Dorfman, R. I., and Shipley, R. A., "Androgens", pp. 119-120, John Wiley and Sons, Inc., New York, N. Y., 1956.

267. Junkman, K., and Witzel, H., Z. Vitamin-, Hormon-Fermentforsch. (1957), 9, 222.

268. Camerino, B., and Sala, G., Progr. Drug Res.
      (1960), 2, 71.
269. Diczfalusy, E., Acta Endocrinol. (1960), 35, 59.
270. Dorner, G., and Shubert, A., Acta Biol. Med. Ger.
      (1963), Suppl. II, 209.
271. Diczfalusy, E., Ferno, O., Fex, H., and Hogberg,
      B., Acta Chem. Scand. (1963), 17, 2536.
272. Dirscherl, W., and Kruskemper, H. L., Biochem.
      Ztschr. (1953), 323, 520.
273. Dekanski, J., and Chapman, R. N., Brit. J. Phar-
      macol. (1953), 8, 271.
274. Kupchan, M., Casy, A. F., and Swintosky, J. V.,
      J. Pharm. Sci. (1965), 54, 514.
275. Lloyd, C. W., and Fredericks, J., J. Clin. Endo-
      crinol. (1951), 11, 724.
276. Ott, A. C., Kuizenga, M. H., Lyster, S. C., and
      Johnson, B. A., J. Clin. Endocrinol. (1952), 12,
      15.
277. Voss, H. E., Arzneim. Forsch. (1955), 5, 208.
278. Haack, E., Stoeck, G., and Voigt, H., Arzneim.
      Forsch. (1955), 5, 211.
279. Deanesly, R., and Parkes, A. S., Biochem. J.
      (1936), 30, 291.
280. Schenk, M., and Junkman, K., Arch. Exp. Path.
      Pharmak. (1955), 227, 210.
281. Dirscherl, W., and Dardenne, U., Biochem. Zschr.
      (1954), 325, 195.
282. Emmens, C. W., Endocrinol. (1941), 28, 633.
283. Kupperman, H. S., Aronson, S. G., Gagliani, J.,
      Parsonnet, M., Roberts, M., Silver, B., and Post-
      iglioni, R., Acta Endocrinol. (1954), 16, 101.
284. Meier, R., and Tschopp, E., Naunyn Schmeidebergs,
      Arch. Exp. Path. Pharmak. (1955), 226, 532.
285. Gould, D., Finckenor, L., Herschberg, E. B.,
      Pearlman, P., Cassidy, J., Margolin, S., and
      Spoerlein, M. T., Chem. Ind. (1955), 1424.
286. Baggett, B., Engel, L. L., Savard, K., and Dorf-
      man, R. I., J. Biol. Chem. (1956), 221, 931.
287. Ruzicka, L., and Kagi, H., Helv. Chim. Acta
      (1936), 19, 842.
288. Sulman, F. G., Horokeach Haivari (1958), 7, 76.
289. Kishimoto, Y., Arch. Biochem. Biophys. (1973),
      159, 528.
290. McEwen, B. S., Pfaff, D. W., and Zigmond, R. E.,
      Brain Res. (1970), 21, 17.
291. Pala, G., Casadio, S., Mantegani, A., Bonardi,
      G., and Coppi, G., J. Med. Chem. (1972), 15, 995.
292. Rapala, R. T., Kraay, R. J., and Gerzon, K., J.
      Med. Chem. (1965), 8, 580.
293. van der Vies, J., Acta Endocrinol. (1965), 49, 271.

294. Chaudry, M. A. Q., and James, K. C., J. Med.
     Chem. (1974), 17, 157.
295. DeVisser, J., and Overbeck, G. A., Acta Endocrin-
     ol. (1960), 35, 405.
296. "American Hospital Formulary Service", American
     Society of Hospital Pharmacists, Washington, D.C.
     (1974), 68, 08.
297. Seay, D. G., Bradshaw, J. D., and Nicol, N. T.,
     Cancer Chemother. Rep. (1972), 56, 89.
298. Kuhl, H., and Taubert, H. D., Steroids (1973),
     22, 73.
299. Diczfalusy, E., and Westman, A., Acta Endocrinol.
     (1956), 21, 321.
300. Falconi, G., Galletti, F., Celasco, G., and
     Gardi, R., Steroids (1972), 20, 627.
301. Ferrin, J., J. Clin. Endocrinol. (1952), 12, 28.
302. Gardi, R., Vitali, R., Falconi, G., and Ercoli,
     A., J. Med. Chem. (1973), 16, 123.
303. Parkes, A. S., J. Endocrinol. (1943), 3, 288.
304. Parkes, A. S., Biochem. J. (1937), 31, 579.
305. Freed, S. C., Eisin, W. M., and Greenhill, J. P.,
     J. Amer. Med. Ass. (1942), 119, 1412.
306. Ferno, O., Fex, H., Hogberg, B., Linderot, T.,
     Veige, S., and Diczfalusy, E., Acta Chem. Scand.
     (1958), 12, 1675.
307. Tillinger, K. G., and Westman, A., Acta Endocrin-
     ol. (1957), 25, 113.
308. American Home Products Co., U. S. Patent
     3,647,784 (March 7, 1972).
309. American Home Products Co., U. S. Patent
     3,649,621 (March 14, 1972).
310. Yamada, J., Toko Igakkai Zasshi (1959), 6, 481.
311. Rizkallah, T. H., and Taymor, M. L., Adv. Planned
     Parenthood Int. Congr. Series (1967), #138, 111.
312. Zartman, E. R., Adv. Planned Parenthood Int.
     Congr. Series (1967), #138, 116.
313. Haspels, A. A., Ned. Tijdschr. Geneesk. (1970),
     114, 61.
314. "American Hospital Formulary Services", American
     Society of Hospital Pharmacists, Washington, D.C.
     (1974), 68, 32.
315. Gross, F., and Tschopp, E., Experientia (1952),
     8, 75.
316. "American Hospital Formulary Service", American
     Society of Hospital Pharmacists, Washington, D.C.
     (1974), 68, 04.
317. Winter, C. A., and Porter, C. C., J. Amer. Pharm.
     Ass. Sci. Ed. (1957), 46, 515.

318. "American Hospital Formulary Service", American Society of Hospital Pharmacists, Washington, D.C. (1974), 28, 16.08.
319. Enerheim, B., Gottfries, C. G., and Sunden, C., Nor. Psyk. Tidskr. (1970), 24, 239.
320. Ebert, A. G., and Hess, S. M., J. Pharmacol. Exp. Ther. (1965), 148, 412.
321. Kincross-Wright, J., and Charalampous, K. D., J. Neuropsychiat. (1965), 1, 66.
322. Mishinsky, J., Khazen, K., and Sulman, F. G., Neuroendocrinol. (1969), 4, 321.
323. Dreyfus, J., Ross, Jr., J. J., and Schreiber, E. C., J. Pharm. Sci. (1971), 60, 829.
324. Denham, J., and Adamson, L., Acta Psychiat. Scand. (1971), 47, 420.
325. Nymark, M., Franck, K. F., Pedersen, V., Boeck, V., and Nielsen, I. M., Acta Pharmacol. Toxicol. (1973), 33, 363.
326. Jørgensen, A., Overø, K. F., and Hansen, V., Acta Pharmacol. Toxicol. (1971), 29, 339.
327. Villeneuve, A., Pires, A., Jus, A., Lachance, R., and Drolet, A., Cur. Ther. Res. (1972), 14, 696.
328. Ayd, F. J., Int. Drug Ther. Newsletter (1972), 7, 1.
329. Villeneuve, A., and Simon, P., J. Ther. (1971), 2, 3.
330. Thomsen, J. B., and Birkerod, D., Acta Psychiat. Scand. (1973), 49, 119.
331. Julou, L., Bourat, G., Ducrot, R., Fournel, J., and Garrett, C., Acta Psychiat. Scand. (1973), 241, 9.
332. Elslager, E. F., Tendick, F. H., and Werbel, L. M., J. Med. Chem. (1969), 12, 600.
333. Elslager, E. F., Progr. Drug Res. (1969), 13, 170.
334. Thompson, P. E., Int. J. Lepr. (1967), 35, 605.
335. Carrington, H. C., Crowther, A. F., Davey, D. G., Levi, A. A., and Rose, F. L., Nature, (1951), 168, 1080.
336. Waitz, J. A., Olszewski, B. J., and Thompson, P. E., Science (1963), 141 723.
337. Ryley, J. F., Brit. J. Pharmacol. (1953), 8, 424.
338. Coatney, G. R., Contacos, P. G., and Lunn, J. S., Amer. J. Trop. Med. Hyg. (1964), 13, 383.
339. Crowther, A. F., and Levi, A. A., Brit. J. Pharmacol. (1953), 8, 93.
340. Carrington, H. C., Crowther, A. F., and Stacey, G. J., J. Chem. Soc. (1954), 1017.
341. Elslager, E. F., and Worth, D. F., Nature (1965), 206, 630.

342. Thompson, P. E., Olszewski, B. J., Elslager, E. F., and Worth, D. F., Amer. J. Trop. Med. Hyg. (1963), 12, 481.

343. Elslager, E. F., Gavrilis, Z. B., Phillips, A. A., and Worth, D. F., J. Med. Chem. (1969), 12, 357.

344. Elslager, E. F., Capps, D. B., and Worth, D. F., J. Med. Chem. (1969), 12, 597.

345. Halpern, A., Shaftel, N., and Bovi, A. J. M., Amer. J. Pharm. (1958), 130, 190.

346. Levine, R. H., Zaks, A., Fink, M., and Freedman, A. (1972), New York Medical College and Metropolitan Hospital Center. See Ref. 241.

347. Caldwell, H. C., Rednick, A. B., Scott, G. C., Yakatan, G. J., and Ziv, D., J. Pharm. Sci. (1970), 59, 1689.

348. Shibini, H. A. M., Nasser, M. A., and Motarvi, M. M., Pharmazie (1971), 26, 630.

349. Gray, A. P., and Robinson, D. S., J. Pharm. Sci. (1974), 63, 159.

350. Gray, A. D., and Robinson, D. S., First International Conference on Narcotic Antagonists, Airlie House, Warrenton, Va., November 1972.

351. Cavallito, C. J., and Jewel, R., J. Amer. Pharm. Assoc. Sci. Ed. (1958), 47, 165.

352. Thomspon, R. E., and Hecht, R. A., Amer. J. Clin. Nutr. (1959), 7, 311.

353. Lawrence, R. D., Brit. Med. J. (1955), 1, 603.

354. Benedetti, M. S., and Larue, D. A., Arzneim. Forsch. (1973), 23, 826.

355. Hinsvark, O. N., Truant, A. P., Jenden, D. J., and Steinborn, J. A., J. Pharmacokin. Biopharm. (1973), 1, 319.

356. Miller, Jr., W. C., Marcotte, D. B., and McCurdy, L., Curr. Ther. Res. (1973), 15, 700.

357. Garrett, T. A., Clin. Med. (1956), 3, 1185.

358. Bundalo, T. S., Fugazzato, D. J., and Wyczalek, J. V., Amer. J. Trop. Med. Hyg. (1969), 18, 50.

359. Haves, H. L., and Lynch, J. E., J. Parasitol. (1967), 53, 1085.

360. Saias, F., Jondet, A., and Phillipe, J., Ann. Pharm. Fr. (1969), 27, 557.

361. Borodkin, S., and Yunker, M. H., J. Pharm. Sci. (1970), 59, 481.

362. Borodkin, S., and Sundberg, D. P., J. Pharm. Sci. (1971), 70, 1523.

363. Loucas, S. P., and Haddad, H. M., J. Pharm. Sci. (1972), 61, 985.

364. Myddleton, W. W., J. Soc. Cosmetic Chem. (1960), 11, 192.

365. Cohen, S., Drug Cosmetic Ind. (1957), 81, 306.
366. Weiner, B. Z., and Zilkha, A., J. Med. Chem. (1973), 16, 573.
367. Garner, D. D., and Garson, L. R., J. Pharm. Sci. (1973), 62, 2049.
368. Greenblatt, D. J., Shader, R. I., and Koch-Wesser, J., N. Engl. J. Med. (1974), 291, 1116.
369. Gamble, J. A. S., MacKay, J. S., and Dundee, J. W., Brit. J. Anaesth. (1973), 45, 926.
370. Gamble, J. A. S., MacKay, J. S., and Dundee, J. W., Brit. J. Anaesth. (1973), 45 1085.
371. Baldwin, J., and Amerson, A. B., Amer. J. Hosp. Pharm. (1973), 30, 837.
372. Rowland, M., "Clinical Pharmacology" p. 27, Macmillan Co., New York, N. Y., 1972.
373. Dam, M., and Olesen, V., Neurol. (1966), 16, 288.
374. Serrano, E. E., Roye, D. B., and Hammer, R. H., Neurol. (1973), 23, 311.
375. Wilensky, A. J., and Lowden, J. A., Neurol. (1973), 23, 318.
376. Lange, W. E., and Stein, M. E., J. Pharm. Sci. (1964), 53, 435.
377. Kawamura, M., Yamamoto, R., and Fujisawa, S., Yakugaku Zasshi. (1971), 91, 879.
378. "The Merck Index", p. 861, Eighth Ed., Stecher, P. G., ed., Merck and Co., Rahway, N. J., 1968.
379. Melby, J. C., and St. Cyr, M., Metabolism (1961), 10, 75.
380. Novak, E., Stabbs, S., and Chodos, D. J., Clin. Pharmacol. Ther. (1972), 13, 148.
381. "The Merck Index", p. 542, Eighth Ed., Stecher, P. G., ed., Merck and Co., Rahway, N. Y., 1968.
382. Yamamoto, R., Fujisawa, S., and Kawamura, M., Yakugaku Zasshi (1971), 91, 855.
383. Kawamura, M., Yamamoto, R., and Fujisawa, S., Yakagaku Zasshi (1971), 91, 863.
384. Kawamura, M., Yamamoto, R., and Fujisawa, S., Yakugaku Zasshi (1971), 91, 871.
385. Flynn, G., and Lamb, D. J., J. Pharm. Sci. (1970) 59, 1433.
386. Kampman, J., Hansen, J. M., Siersbaek-Nielsen, K., and Laursen, H., Clin. Pharmacol. Ther. (1972), 13, 516.
387. Sandman, B., "The Chemistry of Chloramphenicol 3-Monosuccinate", Ph.D. thesis, U. Wisconsin, 1968.
388. Sandman, B., Szulczewski, D., Winheuser, J., and Higuchi, T., J. Pharm. Sci. (1970), 59, 427.
389. Druckrey, H., and Raabe, S., Klin. Wschr. (1952), 30, 882.

390. Brandes, D., and Bourne, G. H., Lancet (1955), 481.
391. Wilmanns, H., Medizinsche (1954), 1, 17.
392. Flocks, R. H., Marberger, H., Begley, B. J., and Prendergast, L. J., J. Urol. (1955), 74, 549.
393. Gadermann, E., Klin. Wschr. (1952), 30, 882.
394. Framondino, M., Marino, G., Randazzo, G., and Scardi, V., Il Farmaco Ed. Sci. (1971), 26, 294.
395. Druckrey, H., Dtsch. Med. Wschr. (1952), 77, 1495.
396. Druckrey, H., Dtsch. Med. Wschr. (1952), 77, 1534.
397. Jacob, H., and Rothauge, C., Zschr. Urol. (1956), 49, 301.
398. "The Merck Index", p. 549-550, Eighth Ed., Stecher, P. G., ed., Merck and Co, Rahway, N. J., 1968.
399. Glazko, A. J., Carnes, H. E., Kazenko, A., Wolf, L. M., and Reutner, T. F., Antibiot. Ann. (1957-1958), 792.
400. Ross, S., Puig, J. R., and Zaremba, E. A., Antibiot. Ann. (1957-1958), 803.
401. Payne, H. M., and Hachney, Jr., R. L., Antibiot. Ann. (1957-1958), 821.
402. McCrumb, Jr., F. R., Snyder, M. J., and Hicken, W. J., Antibiot. Ann. (1957-1958), 837.
403. LePage, G. A., Lin, Y. T., Orth, R. E., and Gottlieb, J. A., Cancer Res. (1972), 32, 2441.
404. Hanessian, S., J. Med. Chem. (1973), 16, 290.
405. Kaplan, S. A., Jack, M. L., Alexander, K., and Weinfeld, R. E., J. Pharm. Sci. (1973), 62, 1789.
406. DeSilva, J. A. F., Koechlin, B. A., and Bader, G., J. Pharm. Sci. (1966), 55, 692.
407. Marcucci, F., Fanelli, R., Mussini, E., and Garattini, S., Europ. J. Pharmacol. (1969), 7, 307.
408. Berlin, A., Sirvers, B., Agurell, S., Hiort, A., Sjöqvist, F., and Ström, S., Clin. Pharmacol. Ther. (1972), 13, 733.
409. Walkenstein, S. S., Wiser, R., Gudmundsen, C. H., Kimmel, H. B., and Corradino, R. A., J. Pharm. Sci. (1964), 53, 1181.
410. Salmona, M., Saronio, C., Bianchi, R., Marcucci, F., and Mussini, E., J. Pharm. Sci. (1974), 63, 222.
411. Pelzer, H., and Maass, D., Arzniem. Forsch. (1969), 6, 1652.
412. Graziani, G., and DeMarchi, F., Boll. Soc. Ital. Biol. Sper. (1967), 43, 1422.

413. Babbini, M., DeMarchi, F., Montanaro, N.,
     Strocchi, P., and Torrielli, M. N., Arzneim.
     Forsch. (1969), 19, 1931.
414. Stella, V., and Higuchi, T., J. Pharm. Sci.
     (1973), 62, 962.
415. Atkinson, Jr., A. J., and Davidson, R., Ann. Rev.
     Med. (1974), 25, 99.
416. "The Merck Index", pp. 652-653, Eighth Ed.,
     Stecher, P. G., ed. Merck and Co., Rahway, N. Y.,
     1968.
417. Greenberg, F. H., Leung, K. K., and Leung, M.,
     J. Chem. Ed. (1971), 48, 632.
418. "American Hospital Formulary Service", American
     Society of Hospital Pharmacists, Washington, D.
     C. (1974), 88, 24.
419. Zitko, B. A., Howes, J. F., Razdan, R. K.,
     Dalzell, H. C., Sheehan, J. C., Pars, H. G.,
     Dewey, W. L., and Harris, L. S., Science (1972),
     179, 442.
420. Little, A. D., U. S. Patent 3,728,360 (April 17,
     1973).
421. Editorial, Chem. Eng. News (1974), Sept. 30,
     15.
422. Marcus, A., U. S. Patent 3,230,143 (1966).
423. Butler, T. C., J. Pharmacol. Exp. Ther. (1952),
     104, 299.
424. Bogue, J. Y., and Carrington, H. C., Brit. J.
     Pharmacol. (1953), 8, 230.
425. Kutt, H., Clin. Pharmacol. Ther. (1974), 16, 243.
426. Husman, J. W., Pharm. Weekbl. (1969), 104, 799.
427. Fujimoto, J. M., Mason, W. H., and Murphy, M.,
     J. Pharmacol. Exp. Ther. (1968), 159, 379.
428. Bogan, J., and Smith, H., J. Pharm. Pharmacol.
     (1968), 20, 64.
429. Arcamone, F., Franceschi, G., Minghetti, A.,
     Denco, S., Redaelli, S., DiMarco, A. D., Casazza,
     A. M., Dasdia, T., DiFronzo, G., Guiliani, F.,
     Lenaz, L., Necco, A., and Soranzo, C., J. Med.
     Chem. (1974), 17, 335.
430. Davenport, H. W., Gastroenerol. (1965), 49, 189.
431. Davenport, H. W., Gastroenterol. (1965), 49, 238.
432. Smith, M. J. H., and Smith, P. K., "The Salicy-
     lates", pp. 235-257, Interscience Pub., New York,
     N. Y., 1966.
433. Stubbé, L. Th. F. L., Pietersen, J. H., and Van
     Heulen, C., Brit. Med. J. (1962), 675.
434. Pierson, R. N., Holt, P. R., Watson, R. M., and
     Keating, R. P., Amer. J. Med. (1961), 31, 259.
435. Menguy, R., Gastroenterol. (1966), 51, 430.

436. Wood, P. H. N., Harvey-Smith, E. A., and Dixon, A. S. J., Brit. Med. J. (1962), 669.

437. Hurst, A., Brit. Med. J. (1943), 768.

438. Leonards, J. P., and Levy, G., J. Pharm. Sci. (1970), 59, 1511.

439. Anderson, K. W., Arch. Int. Pharmacodyn. (1964), 152, 379.

440. Douthwaite, A. H., Lancet (1954), 917.

441. Davenport, H. W., Gastroenterol. (1964), 46, 245.

442. Croft, D. N., Cuddigan, J. H. P., and Sweetland, C., Brit. Med. J. (1972), 545.

443. Misher, A., Adams, H. J., Fishler, J. J., and Jones, R. G., J. Pharm. Sci. (1968), 57, 1128.

444. Dittert, L. W., Caldwell, H. C., Ellison, T., Irwin, G. M., Rivard, D. E., and Swintosky, J. V., J. Pharm. Sci. (1968), 57, 828.

445. Hussain, A., Yamasaki, M., and Truelove, J. E., J. Pharm. Sci. (1974), 63, 627.

446. Schering Corp., U. S. Patent 3,767,811 (Oct. 23, 1973).

447. Kutnowskie Zakay Farmaceutyzine Polfa, French Patent 1,604,123 (Aug. 20, 1971).

448. Bailey, D. M., Wood, D., Johnson, R. E., McAuliff, J. P., Bradford, J. C., and Arnold, A., J. Med. Chem. (1972), 15, 344.

449. Glamkowski, E. J., Gal, G., and Sletzinger, M., J. Med. Chem. (1973), 16, 176.

450. Izquierdo, M., Gomis, P., U. S. Patent 3,607,881 (Sept. 21, 1971).

451. Ludwig, G., and Ache, I. M., Arzneim. Forsch. (1973), 23, 1226.

452. Riedel, R., and Schoetensack, W., Arzneim. Forsch. (1973), 23, 1215.

453. Konig, J., Knoche, C., and Schafer, H., Arzneim. Forsch. (1973), 23, 1246.

454. Benakis, A., Tsoukas, G., and Glasson, B., Arzneim. Forsch. (1973), 23, 1231.

455. Jones, W. G. M., Thorp, J. M. T., and Waring, W. S., (to Imperial Chemical Industries Ltd.) Brit. Patent 860,303 (1961).

456. Barrett, A. M., and Throp, J. M. T., Brit. J. Pharmacol. Chemother. (1968), 32, 381.

457. Klebanov, B. M., Farmakol. Toksikol. (1970), 33, 324. (through Chem. Abstr. 73, 64752m).

458. Beirsdorf, A. G., West Ger. Patent 2,212,830 (Sept. 27, 1973).

459. Beirsdorf, A. G., West Ger. Patent 2,212,831 (Sept. 27, 1973).

460. Novak, E., Wagner, J. G., and Lamb, D. J., Int.
      J. Clin. Pharmacol., Ther. Toxicol. (1970), 3,
      201.
461. Morozowich, W., Lamb, D. J., DeHaan, R. M., and
      Gray, J. E., p. 63, Abstracts of Papers, A.Ph.A.
      Academy of Pharmaceutical Sciences, Washington,
      D. C. Meeting, April 1970.
462. Martin, L. E., Bates, C. M., Beresford, C. R.,
      Donaldson, J. D., McDonald, F. F., Dunlop, D.,
      Sheard, P., London, E., and Twigg, G. D., Brit.
      J. Pharmacol. (1955), 10, 375.
463. Beresford, C. R., Golberg, L., and Smith, J. P.,
      Brit. J. Pharmacol. (1957), 12, 107.
464. Fletcher, F., and London, E., Brit. Med. J.
      (1954), 984.
465. Olsson, K. S., and Weinfeld, A., Acta Med. Scand.
      (1972), 192, 543.
466. Olsson, K. S., Lundvall, O., and Weinfeld, A.,
      Acta Med. Scand. (1972), 191, 49.
467. Olsson, K. S., Acta Med. Scand. (1972), 192, 551.
468. Terato, K., Fujita, T., and Yoshino, Y., J.
      Pharm. Soc. Jap. (1972), 92, 1247.
469. Terato, K., Hiramatsu, Y., and Yoshino, Y., Amer.
      J. Dig. Dis. (1973), 18, 129.
470. Terato, K., Fujita, T., and Yoshino, Y., Amer. J.
      Dig. Dis. (1973), 18, 121.
471. Bonner, D. P., Mechlinski, W., and Schaffner, C.
      P., J. Antibiot. (1972), 25, 261.
472. "The Merck Index", p. 75, Eighth Ed., Stecher, P.
      G., ed. Merck and Co., Rahway, N. J., 1968.
473. Anderson, N. H., and Weinshenker, N. M., U. S.
      Patent 3,723,473 (March 27, 1973).
474. Edgerton, W. H., U. S. Patent 2,662,906 (1953).
475. Glazko, A. J., Edgerton, W. H., Dill, W. A., and
      Lenz, W. R., Antibiot. Chemother. (1952), 2, 234.
476. Siegert, R., and Vömel, W., Anzneim. Forsch.
      (1956), 6, 714.
477. Taylor, E. P., J. Pharm. Pharmacol. (1953), 5,
      254.
478. Houtman, R. L., U. S. Patent 3,447,926 (May 6,
      1969).
479. Sumitomo Chem. Co. Ltd., West Ger. Patent
      2,244,179 (March 29, 1973).
480. Aguiar, A. J., Krc, J., Kinkel, A. W., and Samyn,
      J. C., J. Pharm. Sci. (1967), 56, 847.
481. Glazko, A. J., Dill, W. A., Kazenko, A., Wolf, L.
      M., and Carnes, H. E., Antibiot. Chemother.
      (1958), 8, 516.

482.   Andersgaard, H., Finholt, P., Gjermundsen, R., and Høyland, T., Acta Pharm. Suecica (1974), 11, 239.

483.   Kier, L. B., J. Pharm. Sci. (1972), 61, 1394.

484.   Boncrieff, R. W., "The Chemical Senses", pp. 490-543, Leonard Hill, London, England, 1967.

485.   Kubota, T., and Kubo, I., Nature (1969), 223, 97.

486.   Jones, P. H., Rowley, E. K., Weiss, A. L., Bishop, D. L., and Chun, A. H. C., J. Pharm. Sci. (1969), 58, 337.

487.   Morozowich, W., Sinkula, A. A., MacKellar, F. A., and Lewis, C., J. Pharm. Sci. (1973), 62, 1102.

488.   Sinkula, A. A., and Lewis, C., J. Pharm. Sci. (1973), 62, 1757.

489.   Morozowich, W., Sinkula, A. A., Karnes, H. A., MacKellar, F. A., Lewis, C., Stern, K. F., and Rowe, E. L., J. Pharm. Sci. (1969), 58, 1485.

490.   Celmer, C. D., Canad. Patent 779,315 (Feb. 27, 1968).

491.   "American Hospital Formulary Service", American Society of Hospital Pharmacists, Washington, D.C. (1974), 8, 24.

492.   Officina Terapeutica Italiana Srl, French Patent 2,099,449 (Mar. 17, 1972).

493.   Repta, A. J., and Hack, J., J. Pharm. Sci. (1973), 62, 1892.

494.   Dittert, L. W., Caldwell, H. C., Adams, H. J., Irwin, G. M., and Swintosky, J. V., J. Pharm. Sci. (1968), 57, 774.

495.   Dittert, L. W., Irwin, G. M., Chong, C. W., and Swintosky, J. V., J. Pharm. Sci. (1968), 57, 780.

496.   Rattie, E. S., Shami, E. G., Dittert, L. W., and Swintosky, J. V., J. Pharm. Sci. (1970), 59, 1738.

497.   Swintosky, J. V., Caldwell, H. C., Chong, C. W., Dittert, L. W., and Irwin, G. M., J. Pharm. Sci. (1968), 57, 752.

498.   Swintosky, J. V., Adams, H. J., Caldwell, H. C., Dittert, L. W., Ellison, T., and Rivard, D. E., J. Pharm. Sci. (1966), 55, 992.

499.   Rice, W. B., and McColl, J. W., J. Amer. Pharm. Assoc. Sci. Ed. (1956), 45, 137.

500.   Butler, T. C., J. Pharmacol. Exp. Ther. (1948), 92, 49.

501.   Editorial, Drug Intel. Clin. Pharm. (1973), 7, 126.

502.   Caldwell, H. C., Adams, H. J., Rivard, D. E., and Swintosky, J. V., J. Pharm. Sci. (1967), 56, 920.

503. "American Hospital Formulary Service", American
      Society of Hospital Pharmacists, Washington, D.C.
      (1974), 8, 08.
504. "American Hospital Formulary Service", American
      Society of Hospital Pharmacists, Washington, D.C.
      (1974), 28, 16.08.
505. "American Hospital Formulary Service", American
      Society of Hospital Pharmacists, Washington, D.C.
      (1974), 56, 20.
506. Gruber, Jr., C. M., Stephens, V. C., and Terrill,
      P. M., Toxicol. Appl. Pharmacol. (1971), 19, 423.
507. Emmerson, J. L., Gibson, W. R., and Anderson, R.
      C., Toxicol. Appl. Pharmacol. (1971), 19, 445.
508. Wolen, R. L., Gruber, Jr., C. M., Kiplinger, G.
      F., and Scholz, N. F., Toxicol. Appl. Pharmacol.
      (1971), 19, 480.
509. Stephens, V. C., U. S. Patent 3,728,379 (Apr. 17,
      1973).
510. Shapira, F., Adv. Cancer Res. (1973), 18, 77.
511. Wechter, W. J., J. Med. Chem. (1967), 10, 762.
512. Smith, C. G., Buskirk, H. H., and Lumis, W. L.,
      J. Med. Chem. (1967), 10, 774.
513. Fabrica de Medicamente Biofarm. West Ger. Patent
      2,231,486 (Feb. 15, 1973).
514. "American Hospital Formulary Service", American
      Society of Hospital Pharmacists, Washington, D.C.
      (1974), 8, 24.
515. Bruzzese, T., Gio, A., and Riva, M., Il Farm. Ed.
      Sci. (1972), 28, 121.
516. Hubacher, M. H., and Doernberg, S., J. Pharm.
      Sci. (1964), 53, 1067.
517. "The Merck Index", pp. 940-941, Eighth Ed.,
      Stecher, P. G., ed., Merck and Co., Rahway, N. Y.,
      1968.
518. Sokoloski, T. D., and Higuchi, T., J. Pharm. Sci.
      (1962), 51, 172.
519. Higuchi, T., and Schroeter, L. C., J. Amer. Chem.
      Soc. (1960), 82, 1904.
520. Riegelman, S., and Fischer, E. Z., J. Pharm. Sci.
      (1962), 51, 206.
521. Nomura, H., and Sugimoto, K., Chem. Pharm. Bull.
      (1966), 14, 1039.
522. Nomura, H., Kuwayama, M., Ishiguro, T., and Mori-
      moto, S., Chem. Pharm. Bull. (1971), 19, 341.
523. Nomura, H., Shimomura, M., and Morimoto, S.,
      Chem. Pharm. Bull. (1971), 19, 1433.
524. Cutolo, E., and Larizza, A., Gazz. Chim. Ital.
      (1961), 91, 964.

525. Seib, P. A., Liang, Y. T., Lee, C. H., Hoseney, C., and Deyoe, C. W., J. Chem. Soc. Perkin I (1974), 1220.

526. Pitman, I. H., Higuchi, T., Alton, M., and Wiley, R., J. Pharm. Sci. (1972), 61, 918.

527. Guillory, J. K., and Higuchi, T., J. Pharm. Sci. (1962), 51, 100.

528. Forlano, A. J., Jarowski, C. I., and Hammer, H. F., J. Pharm. Sci. (1968), 57, 1184.

529. Forlano, A. J., Jarowski, C. I., Hammer. H. F., and Merritt, E. G., J. Pharm. Sci. (1970), 59, 121.

530. Forlano, A. J., J. Pharm. Sci. (1971), 60, 616.

531. Davies, G. E., and Driver, G. W., Nature (1958), 182, 664.

532. Davies, G. E., Driver, G. W., Hoggarth, E., Martin, A. R., Paige, M. F. C., Rose, F. L., and Wilson, B. R., Brit. J. Pharmacol. (1956), 11, 351.

533. Davies, G. E., and Driver, G. W., Brit. J. Pharmacol. (1957), 12, 434.

534. "American Hospital Formulary Service", American Society of Hospital Pharmacists, Washington, D.C. (1974), 28, 20.

535. Tréfouél, J., Tréfouél, J., Nitti, F., and Bovet, D., Comp. Rend. Soc. Biol. (1935), 120, 756.

536. Brodie, B. B., and Axelrod, J., J. Pharmacol. Exp. Ther. (1949), 97, 58.

537. Brodie, B. B., and Axelrod, J., J. Pharmacol. Exp. Ther. (1948), 94, 29.

538. Flinn, F. B., and Brodie, B. B., J. Pharmacol. Exp. Ther. (1948), 94, 76.

539. Burns, J. J., Rose, R. K., Goodwin, S., Reichenthal, J., Horning, E., and Brodie, B. B., J. Pharmacol. Exp. Ther. (1955), 113, 9.

540. Burns, J. J., Yu, T. F., Berger, L., and Gutmann, A., Amer. J. Med. (1958), 25, 401.

541. Conney, A. H., Trousof, N., and Burns, J. J., J. Pharmacol. Exp. Ther. (1960), 128, 333.

542. Berger, F. M., J. Pharmacol. Exp. Ther. (1952), 104, 229.

543. Berger, F. M., J. Pharmacol. Exp. Ther. (1952), 104, 468.

544. Editorial, J. Amer. Med. Ass. (1961), 175, 388.

545. Freundt, K. J., Arznein. Forsch. (1973), 23, 949.

2

Application of the Pro-drug Approach to Antibiotics

A. A. SINKULA

Research Laboratories, The Upjohn Co., Kalamazoo, Mich. 49001

Antibiotics constitute a valuable adjunct to the physicians therapeutic armamentarium in the battle against a wide variety of infectious diseases. While many antibiotics can be utilized with a minimum of modification to ensure their therapeutic effect, exceptions exist where extensive development must be undertaken prior to their becoming efficacious medicinal agents. Certain shortcomings of these agents, such as lack of stability or poor bioavailability,can be minimized or eliminated by the use of carefully designed dosage formulations. In many instances, however, formulation development fails to improve those properties of the antibiotic that are necessary to ensure therapeutic efficacy. It is in this area that chemical modification (prodrug formation) of the parent antibiotic molecule plays an important role.

In the rational design and synthesis of the ideal antibiotic prodrug derivative, several factors should be considered and can be briefly stated as follows:

1. Availability of inexpensive chemical intermediates - any potential derivative should not substantially enhance production costs of an already expensive drug. Most starting materials (acid chlorides or anhydrides, alkyl halides, alkyl or aryl amines, semicarbazides, etc.) considered as chemical modifiers are commercially available in a high state of purity at reasonable costs. Bulk rates are sometimes available on large quantities of certain starting materials thus further lowering overall costs.

2. Derivative easily synthesized and purified - elaborate synthetic schemes should be avoided if at all possible due to increased costs. Multi-step syntheses increase operator time, decrease yields of ultimate product, and increase the probability of unwanted side reactions occurring. Purification should ideally be effected by crystallization from the reaction mixture. Cumbersome separations such as column or liquid chromatography, counter-current distribution, etc., should be avoided when feasible.

3. <u>Derivative conveniently scaled-up in high yield</u> - scale-up problems increase in intensity as a function of the bench scale synthesis. The simpler the bench scale scheme, the less involved are the scale-up problems.

4. <u>Derivative stable in bulk form and in dosage form</u> - many drug derivatives lack a market due to their instability in bulk or dosage form. Such problems as polymorphic changes, degradation in the presence of trace amounts of moisture or solvate, photo-decomposition, caking, melt back, and incompatibilities with vehicle, excipients, lubricants, etc., are common among drug substances. The ideal drug derivative exhibits sufficient physicochemical stability in the bulk and formulated state.

5. <u>Derivative is sufficiently labile in vivo</u> - regeneration of the parent drug molecule <u>in vivo</u> is of essence. The merit of the derivative portion of the drug molecule resides in its ability to modify some undesirable pharmaceutical (physicochemical) property of the parent molecule. It can alter the transport, distribution, site localization, metabolism or excretion characteristics of the parent molecule. Other modifications can include increased solubility (increased bioavailability, decreased pain on injection), decreased solubility (elimination of bitterness or tartness, increased depot bioavailability, increased product stability, decreased gastric or intestinal irritation). For whatever purpose the drug derivative is used, the parent molecule must be regenerated either chemically (pH effects) and/or enzymatically <u>in vivo</u>. In most cases, chemically blocking a functional group of a drug molecule renders the drug therapeutically inactive, thus, the necessity for <u>in vivo</u> lability.

Examples of ensuring <u>in vivo</u> lability of a drug derivative include (a) the use of "activated" esters, e.g. electron withdrawing groups adjacent to the ester bond such as halogens, $-NH_2$, $-NO_2$, ―⟨⟩― R (R=electron withdrawing substituent) and (b) avoidance of steric bulk (t-butyl, i-butyl, i-propyl, etc.) at or near the site of hydrolysis.

6. <u>Derivative is non-toxic</u> - an extremely important consideration in view of the increased toxicological testing required for any and all new promising drug derivatives. Relatively "safe" moieties include amino acids, short to medium length alkyl esters, and many inorganic and organic acid and base salt combinations.

7. <u>The derivative exhibits some real advantage over the parent molecule</u> - prodrug derivatives, by virtue of their ability to clearly modify some pharmaceutical property of a drug substance, make this a fruitful area of drug research. Advantages such as increased absorption and increased serum levels of parent drug, lack of pain on injection, and sustained bioactivity (depot effect) can be claimed. It should be noted that the modification of one property frequently alters several properties of the drug molecule and caution must be exercised when embarking on a program of this nature.

Employing the aforementioned factors as a foundation for our rationale, prodrug derivatives of selected classes of antibiotics will be discussed with emphasis on their chemistry and biology. When pertinent, specific examples will be chosen that illustrate the rationale most emphatically.

β-Lactam Antibiotics

Penicillins.

Ampicillin. Ampicillin (d-α-aminobenzylpenicillin, 1) is a broad-spectrum antibiotic currently enjoying wide use in anti-bacterial therapy against a variety of susceptible gram-positive organisms. While 1 is relatively stable at stomach pH, it is inefficiently absorbed when administered orally.

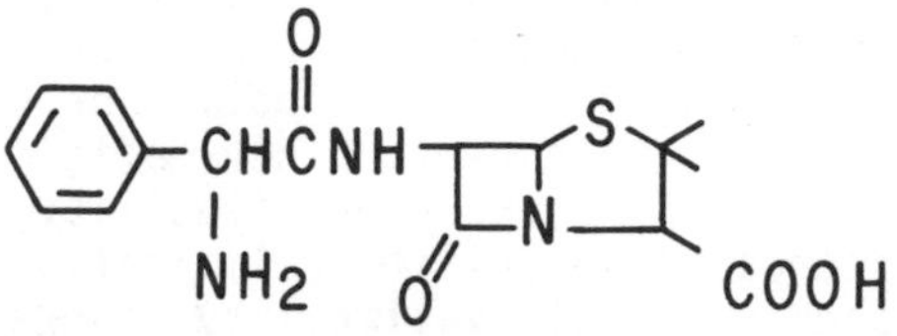

$$\underline{1}$$

Chemistry. In an effort to overcome this absorption problem, von Daehne et.al. (1) prepared a series of acyloxymethyl esters of this antibiotic. In general, two pathways were utilized to prepare a variety of such esters (Scheme I). The first route involves the reaction of potassium benzylpenicillinate 2 with chloromethyl pivalate to form pivaloyloxymethyl benzylpenicillinate 3, followed by hydrolysis of the amide side chain with PCl_5/ quinoline to afford pivaloyloxymethyl 6-aminopenicillinate 4. Treatment of 4 hydrochloride with D-α-phenylglycyl chloride hydrochloride in the presence of sodium bicarbonate gives pivaloyloxymethyl D-α-aminobenzylpenicillinate 5 (pivampicillin) in good yield. 5 was also prepared from 4 by utilizing a β-dicarbonyl protective group approach. A mixed anhydride 6 was prepared by treatment of potassium N-{1-methyl-2-carbethoxyvinyl}-D-α-amino-α-phenylacetate hemihydrate with isobutyl chloroformate. The addition of 4 to a solution of the mixed anhydride afforded the addition product 7 which was hydrolyzed with HCl in situ to give a 65% yield of 5.

The third pathway involves the use of potassium D-α-azido-benzylpenicillinate 8 with formation of the ester 9 by treatment with chloromethyl pivalate. The azide was catalytically hydrogenerated to 5.

Biological. Although pivampicillin is stable in neutral
solution, it is rapidly hydrolyzed to ampicillin in the presence
of esterases derived from a variety of mammalian sources (2).
Esterases obtained from rodent sources, e.g. rat and mouse, exhibit a high degree of hydrolytic activity while esterase enzymes
of dog and man show a somewhat lower activity. Table I summarizes
the in vitro enzyme hydrolysis studies conducted with pivampicillin.

These studies, while indicative of the fate of the ester in
serum and whole blood, do not provide conclusive proof that the
same ester will behave similarly in the intact organism. Human
subjects dosed, in a crossover experiment, with 250 mg. of ampicillin and 358 mg. of pivampicillin (≈250 mg. of ampicillin)
showed absorption of the ester to be equivalent to peak serum
concentrations of ampicillin (after intramuscular injection).
The ester was absorbed almost quantitatively (a three-fold increase in peak serum levels when administered as the ester). It
was further noted that 99% of the drug in blood was present as
ampicillin 15 minutes after administration. Speculation centered
on the fact that, due to the inherent lability of the pivaloyloxymethyl ester, hydrolysis in vivo proceeded via Sequence I.
After absorption of the ester, hydrolysis to the hydroxymethyl
ester occurred followed by further degradation to ampicillin and
formaldehyde.

Hetacillin. Hetacillin {6-(2,2-dimethyl-5-oxo-4-phenyl-1-
imidazolidinyl) penicillanic acid} 11 represents another type of
prodrug of ampicillin (3).

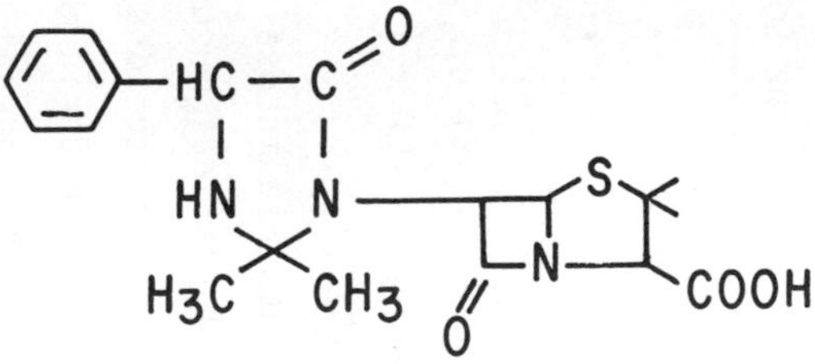

11

This antibiotic derivative was prepared by the condensation of
acetone with ampicillin and was originally designed to enhance
the gastrointestinal absorption of ampicillin. It is also utilized as a stable form of ampicillin for use in infusion solutions
for administration over extended periods of time.

Chemistry. Several methods have been devised whereby 11 can
be prepared from commercially available intermediates (Scheme II).

TABLE I

ENZYMATIC HYDROLYSIS OF PIVAMPICILLIN

Enzyme Source	Half-life[a] (min)
None	103
Mouse serum, 1%	<1
Rat serum, 1%	<1
Dog serum, 5%	50
Dog serum, 10%	23
Human serum, 10%	50
Homogenate of gastric mucosa from the dog, 10%	10
Homogenate of intestinal mucosa from the dog, 10%	5
Liver homogenate from the dog, 10%	<5
Homogenate of human gastric mucosa, 10%	5
Homogenate of human duodenal mucosa, 10%	5
Human whole blood.	5
Whole blood from the dog	3-4

[a]In all experiments, the starting concentration of pivampicillin hydrochloride was 14.3 μg/ml. Determinations were made at pH 7.4 and 37°C. (2)

ANTIMICROBIAL AGENTS AND CHEMOTHERAPY

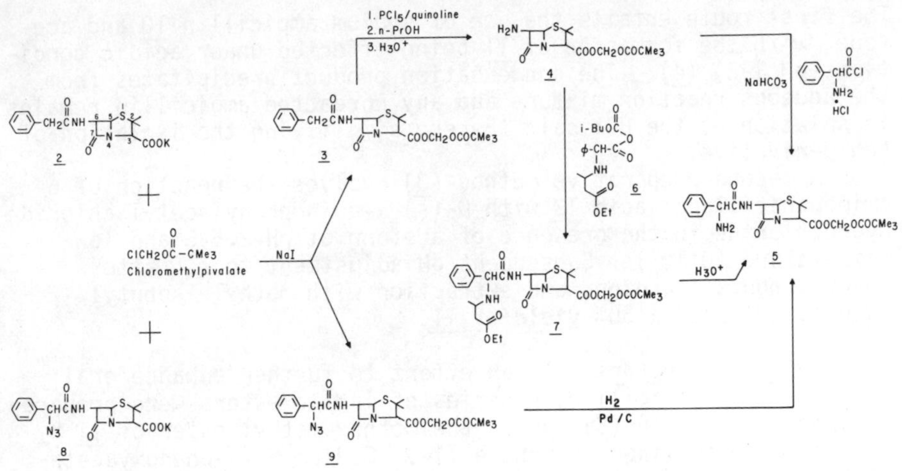

Scheme I

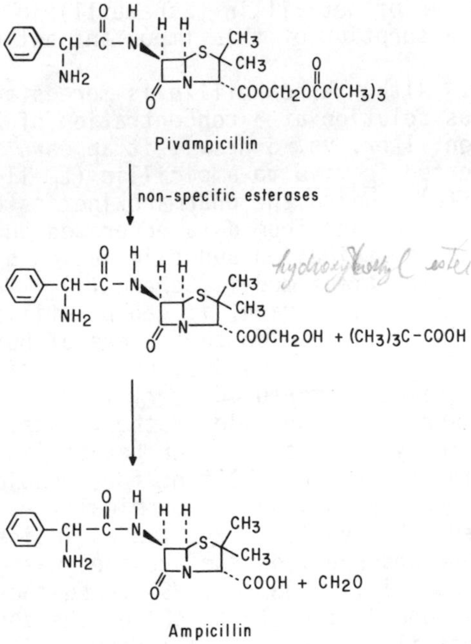

Pivampicillin

non-specific esterases

hydroxybody C ester

Ampicillin

Antimicrobial Agents and Chemotherapy

Sequence I. Hydrolysis of pivampicillin (2)

The first route entails the use of sodium ampicillin 10 and acetone, with the formation of 11 being effected under acidic condi-
tions(pH 1-3) (4). The condensation product precipitates from
the aqueous reaction mixture and any unreacted ampicillin remains
in solution as the HCl salt thereby simplifying the isolation of
the derivative.

A second preparative method (3)involves the reaction of 6-
aminopenicillanic acid 12 with D-(-)-α-aminophenylacetyl chloride
hydrochloride in the presence of acetone at pH 2.5-3 and low
temperature (0-10⁰). Subsequent pH adjustment to 7.5 after
several hours standing, and extraction with methyl isobutyl
ketone, afforded a 50% yield of 11.

Hetacillin esters. In an effort to further enhance oral
absorption of hetacillin, a series of labile esters were prepared.
Sleezer and Johnson (5) formed the methoxymethyl ester of 11 by
the sequence outlined in Scheme III. Sodium 6-(α-phenoxyaceta-
mido) penicillinate 13 was esterified at the C_3 carboxyl with
methoxymethyl chloride and subsequently deacylated at C_6 using
either chemical or enzymatic means to afford methoxymethyl-6-
aminopenicillinate 14. The methoxymethyl ester of ampicillin 15
was produced by reacting 14 with D-(-)-α-aminophenylacetyl
chloride hydrochloride. Condensation of 15 with acetone, under
conditions described previously, afforded a good yield of methoxymethyl hetacillin 16. Essery (6) has similarly prepared the pivaloyloxymethyl ester of hetacillin (Scheme II) in a further effort
to enhance oral absorption of this important antibiotic.

Biological. Although hetacillin is more stable than ampicillin in aqueous solution at a concentration of 250 mg./ml.
(<10% degradation, 1 hr. vs. 6 hrs.), it appears that hetacillin
is rapidly converted in vivo to ampicillin ($t_\frac{1}{2}$ 11±2 minutes) (7).
Jusko and Lewis (8) studied the pharmacokinetics of hetacillin
and ampicillin in man, and from data generated during the study
have described the distribution and elimination of this antibiotic using a two compartment model (Scheme IV). While the model
is perhaps an oversimplification, it can be utilized to quantify
the distribution and elimination parameters of both ampicillin
and hetacillin after intravenous dosing. Table II illustrates
that for those parameters measured, very little, if any, difference exists between the magnitude of the values.

The half-life hydrolysis rate for hetacillin in vivo
averages 11.2 minutes (range 8-13 min. for 8 subjects) and it was
speculated that hydrolysis might be chemically rather than enzymatically mediated. Bioavailability studies indicated that the
amount of the dose absorbed, on the average, was greater for
hetacillin than ampicillin (38% vs. 29%). Further, ampicillin
absorption was enhanced slightly to 42% of the dose when administered as hetacillin during food intake but the reason for
this increased absorption is not apparent.

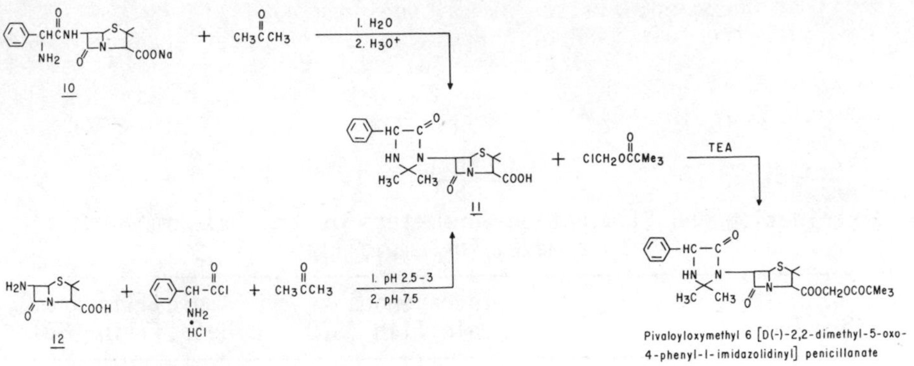

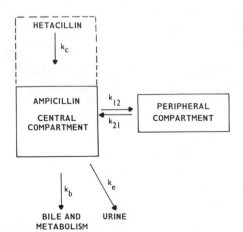

Scheme II

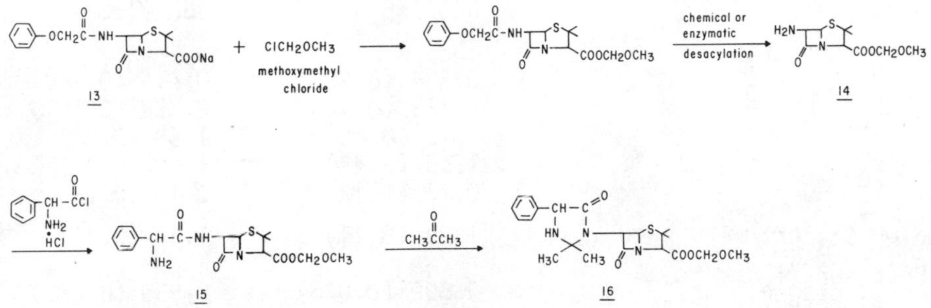

Scheme III

Journal of Pharmaceutical Sciences

Scheme IV. Multiple-compartment pharmacokinetic model used to characterize hetacillin conversion to ampicillin (k_c), ampicillin distribution (k_{12}, k_{21}), and ampicillin renal (k_e) and extrarenal (k_b) elimination (8)

HETACILLIN

k_c

AMPICILLIN CENTRAL COMPARTMENT

k_{12} k_{21}

PERIPHERAL COMPARTMENT

k_b   k_e

BILE AND METABOLISM   URINE

TABLE II

Distribution and Elimination Parameters of the Two-Compartment Open Model for Ampicillin

Parameter[a]	Intravenous Ampicillin (SD)	Ampicillin from Hetacillin (SD)
Distribution volumes, l.		
V_c	12.0 (1.9)	12.5 (2.8)
$V_D ss$	17.9 (1.5)	19.3 (2.9)
Clearances, ml./min.		
Cl_R	341 (91)	296 (91)
Cl_B	335 (56)	350 (102)
Rate constants, hr.$^{-1}$		
k_{12}	0.384 (0.185)	0.419 (0.180)
k_{21}	0.733 (0.163)	0.728 (0.161)
k_{el}	1.73 (0.49)	1.68 (0.30)
k_e	1.55 (0.47)	1.58 (0.31)
k_b	0.17 (0.12)	0.10 (0.13)
Slow $t_{1/2}$, hr.	1.29 (0.11)	1.34 (0.20)
Fraction (f_e) excreted in urine	0.899 (0.075)	0.939 (0.076)
Plasma level area, mcg. hr. ml.$^{-1}$	22.7 (5.2)	22.9 (7.6)
Integral coefficients, hr.		
D_{1a}	0.581 (0.133)	0.581 (0.118)
D_2	0.297 (0.081)	0.355 (0.102)
D_T	0.878 (0.151)	0.921 (0.141)

JOURNAL OF PHARMACEUTICAL SCIENCES

[a] V_c, $V_D ss$, Cl_B, Cl_R, and area are normalized for 1.73 m.^{2} body surface area. (8).

Carbenicillin. Carbenicillin (α-carboxybenzylpenicillin) 17
is an important penicillin analog having unique bioactivity
against pseudomonas aeruginosa and indole-positive Proteus species
which are usually resistant to ampicillin. Carbenicillin is
usually administered parenterally due to its poor gastrointestinal
absorption characteristics. Additionally, it is rendered inactive in the gastric contents due to its acid lability. Many
derivatives, primarily esters, of this antibiotic have been prepared in an attempt to overcome these shortcomings inherent in
the parent molecule.

$$
\underset{\text{CO}_2\text{H}}{\overset{\displaystyle \text{O}}{\underset{\displaystyle}{\text{CH}-\overset{\parallel}{\text{C}}-\text{NH}}}}\qquad \text{CO}_2\text{H}
$$

17

The ester most widely studied to date is carbenicillin indanyl sodium - sodium 6-{2-phenyl-2-(5-indanyloxycarbonyl)}
acetamido penicillinate 19.

Chemistry. The synthesis of 19 is outlined in Scheme V and
was devised by Hobbs (9) as a radiosynthesis utilizing ^{3}H labeled
indanol. The monoacid chloride of phenylmalonic acid was prepared
by treatment of phenylmalonic acid with thionyl chloride in re-
fluxing dimethylformamide. The acid chloride was condensed with
indanol to yield the indanyl ester of phenylmalonic acid 18 in 70%
yield. The acid chloride of 18 was prepared by addition of
thionyl chloride and was subsequently treated with 6-aminopeni-
cillanic acid to afford 19.
        A series of 3-acyloxyalkyl esters was synthesized by Butler
and Hamanaka (10) as labile, lipophilic derivatives of carbenicillin designed to enhance the oral absorption of carbenicillin.
To produce the 3-mono(α-acetoxyethyl) ester 21, α-chloroethyl
acetate is added to a suspension of 6-aminopenicillanic acid 12
(as the triethylamine salt) and stirred for several hours.
(Scheme VI) This ester 20 can be isolated and stored for future
use as the p-toluenesulfonic acid salt or it can be converted
directly to 21 by acylation with phenylmalonic acid mono acid
chloride. This last step in the reaction sequence proceeds
optimally in a heterogeneous solvent system employing water and a
water immiscible inert solvent such as isopropyl ether or benzene
at ice-bath temperature. As the product forms, it partitions
into the organic layer and can be dried and recovered in high
yields.

α-{Carbo(α-acetoxyethyloxy)} benzylpenicillanic acid 21a can
be prepared directly by acylation of 12 with α-acetoxyethyl
phenylmalonyl chloride 22 (11). (Scheme VII). This reaction step
is facilitated by employing a 20-40% molar excess of acid chloride
in a heterogeneous solvent system at a pH of 5.5 - 6.5.

Bis esters of carbenicillin 24 have ideally been made by
direct esterification of carbenicillin disodium salt 23 with the
desired α-acyloxyalkyl halide (Scheme VIII).

Biological. In vitro - the minimal inhibitory concentration
(MIC) of carbenicillin indanyl sodium was determined by a serial
dilution technique using a variety of bacterial isolates of
clinical origin (12). The MIC was found to be similar to carbenicillin but may be misleading since the conditions of the
assay (incubation at 37° C. for 20 hours, alkaline pH conditions)
could cause hydrolysis of the indanyl ester of carbenicillin.

Stability in acidic media. Acid stability is reputedly one
of the major advantages of carbenicillin esters. Studies designed to test this premise were performed by incubating the indanyl ester in synthetic gastric juice (pH2) at 37° C. for one
hour. There was no loss of activity (reflecting acid stability)
for carbenicillin indanyl sodium 19 while disodium carbenicillin
23 lost 99.2% of its antibacterial activity.

Carbenicillin indanyl ester is the derivative that has
been studied most intensively in several mammalian species (9).
In rats, absorption of 19 is virtually quantitative. Using radio
labeled indanyl carbenicillin, >99% of the dose is excreted via
the urine in 24 hours. Only traces of radioactivity are found in
the feces indicating that this ester derivative greatly enhances
absorption of carbenicillin. The ester is rapidly hydrolyzed
after absorption and the labeled indanol is excreted as the
glucuronide and sulfate conjugates. Using the dog as the biological model for absorption studies, the absorption and excretion patterns are more complex. Assay of dog urine after administration of indanyl carbenicillin indicate that about 20% of the
dose presented as indanol conjugates. The remainder appear as
other conjugated metabolites of indanol (Scheme IX) in the form
of hydroxy indanols and hydroxy indanones.

Bioavailability studies carried out with 12 human volunteers,
who were administered a single one gram dose, paralleled the absorption and excretion pattern found in rats (9). Thus, that
amount of indanol (as the glucuronide and sulfate conjugates)
theoretically attributable to the amount of ester administered
was accounted for in the urine. The indanyl ester appears to be
rapidly absorbed quantitatively from the gastrointestinal tract
with subsequent hydrolysis by non-specific serum and tissue
esterases to carbenicillin.

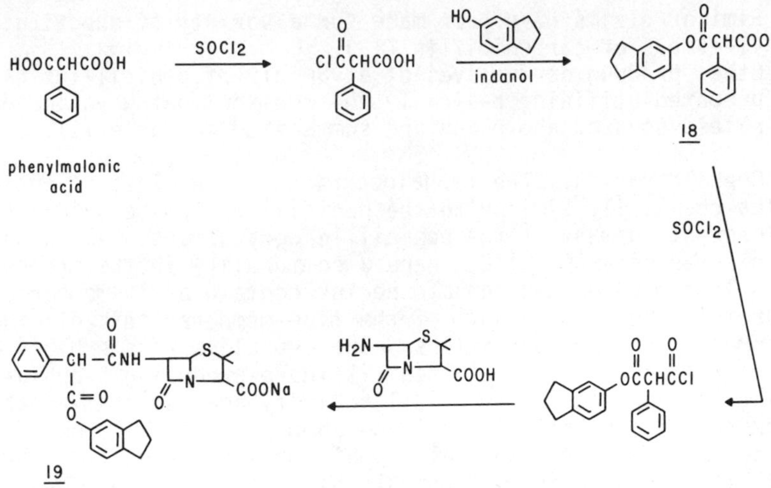

Scheme V

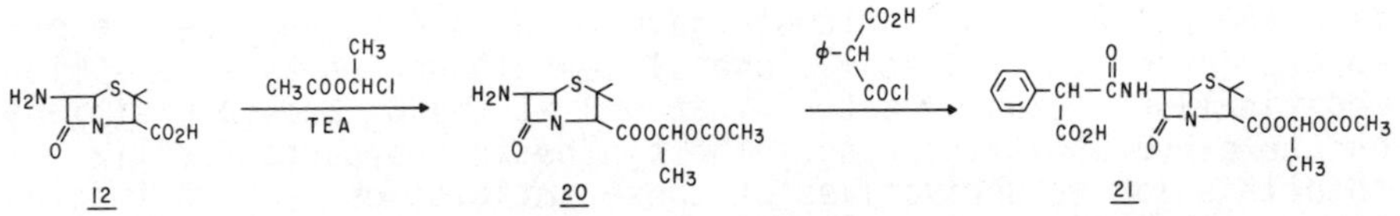

Scheme VI

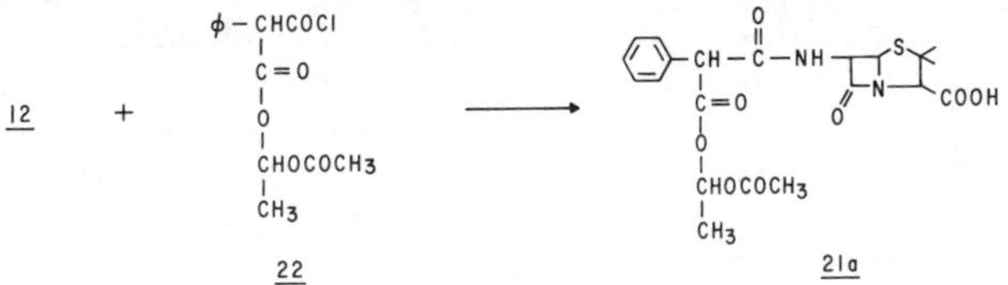

Scheme VII

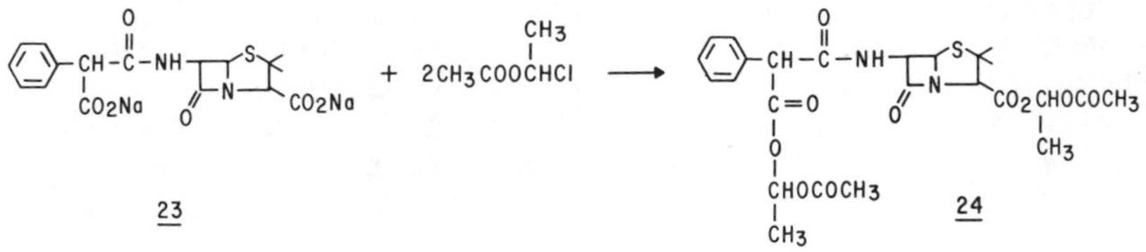

Scheme VIII

Similar claims have been made for a variety of substituted thienyl esters of carbenicillin (13).

Other prodrug derivatives of a variety of penicillins have been prepared utilizing basically the chemical pathways and rationale discussed above and are summarized in Table III.

Cephalosporins. The cephalosporins, a new class of antibiotics chemically similar to the penicillins, possess advantages not inherent in many of the penicillin derivatives. Although both classes of antibiotics share a commonality in the presence of a β-lactam ring, the cephalosporins contain a six-membered dihydrothiazine ring in lieu of the five-membered thiazolidine ring present in the penicillins. The cephalosporins exhibit a high degree of resistance to penicillinase-producing staphlococci (35), possess bactericidal activity against gram-negative and gram-positive bacteria (36) and show no cross-allergenicity with penicillin (37). Several cephalosporins currently enjoying clinical acceptance include cephalothin, cephaloridine, cephaloglycin and cephalexin.

Despite the fact that the cephalosporins exhibit adequate stability in acidic media, they are poorly absorbed on oral administration. Cephaloglycin and cephalexin, however, have demonstrated higher serum levels than cephalothin and cephaloridine (38-41). Various attempts have been made to enhance the oral absorption of the clinically useful cephalosporins by reversible modifications (usually esterification) at the C_3 and C_4 positions on the dihydrothiazine ring. The synthetic approaches utilized to obtain labile derivatives of these antibiotics is both imaginative and voluminous and an effort will be made here only to highlight some of the more successful accomplishments. Specific examples will be used throughout the discussion.

Chemistry - C_3 esters (cephalothin). The achievements of Flynn (42) and Kukolja (43,44) exemplify the unique synthetic routes taken to obtain C_3 esters. The initial step involves the preparation of 7-(2'-thienylacetamido)-3-hydroxymethyl-Δ^2-cephem-4-carboxylic acid 26 by the simultaneous hydrolysis and isomerization of 7-(2'-thienylacetamido) cephalosporanic acid (cephalothin, 25) with sodium hydroxide. (Scheme X). 26 was then esterified with cyclobutane carboxylic anhydride in pyridine to yield 7-(2'thienylacetamido)-3-cyclobutylcarbonyloxymethyl-Δ^2-cephem-4-carboxylic acid 27. Isomerization to the Δ^3 ester was accomplished by warming equimolar quantities of 27 and m-chloroperbenzoic acid for 10 minutes. Isolation of 7-(2'-thienyl-acetamido)-3-cyclobutylcarbonyloxymethyl-Δ^3-cephem-1-oxide-4-carboxylic acid 28 as crystals was achieved by evaporating the majority of the solvent. Reduction of the 1-oxide with stannous chloride and acetyl chloride yielded 7-(2'thienylacetamido)-3-cyclobutylcarbonyloxymethyl-Δ^3-cephem-4-carboxylic acid 29.

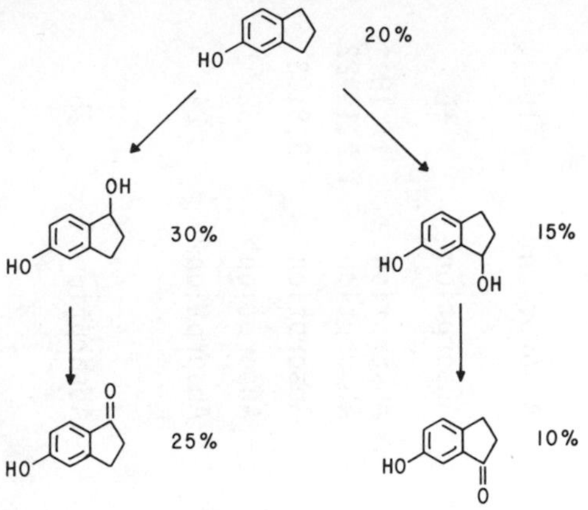

Antimicrobial Agents and Chemotherapy

Scheme IX. Indanol metabolites in dog urine after administration of indanol or indanyl carbenicillin. The figures represent the relative amounts of each substance present. All are present in urine as their glucuronide and sulfate ester conjugates (9).

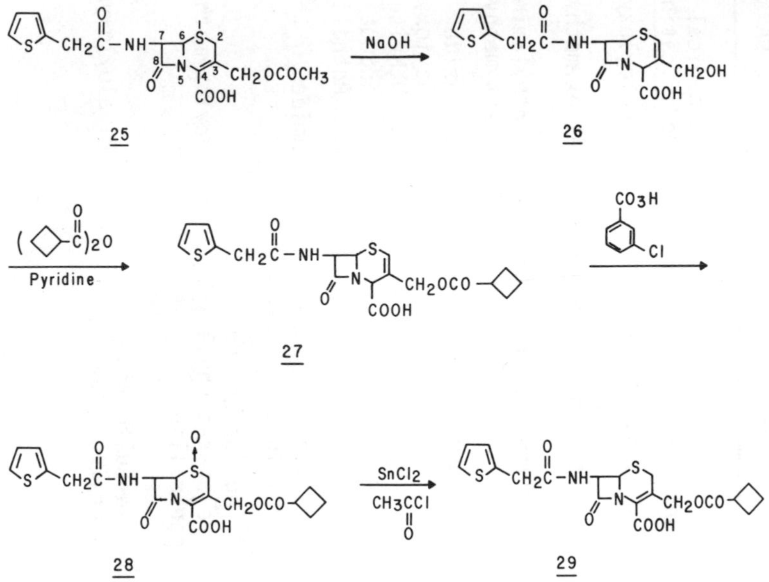

Scheme X

TABLE III. PENICILLIN PRODRUGS DESIGNED TO MODIFY VARIOUS PROPERTIES
OF THE PARENT ANTIBIOTIC

	Parent Molecule	Chemical Modification	Route of Administration	Property Modified	Reference
1.	6-N'-Cyanoamidopenicillin	Pivaloyloxymethyl ester	Oral	Absorption	14
2.	α-Aryl-β-aminoethylpenicillin	Alkoxymethyl esters	Oral	Absorption	15
3.	Penicillin, general structure	Diethylaminoethyl esters, alkoxymethyl esters, ether	Oral	Absorption	16
4.	α-Aminobenzyl penicillin	a. Azide	Oral, IV	Absorption	17,18
		b. Acyloxymethyl esters	Oral	Absorption	1,2,19-22
		c. N,N-isopropylidene adduct	Oral	Absorption	3,8,23
		d. Phthalidyl ester	Oral	Absorption	32
5.	Penicillin G Penicillin V	Amide	IM	Absorption	24
6.	α-Amino (or ureido) cyclohexadienylalkyl penicillin	Acyloxymethyl esters	Oral	Absorption	25
7.	6-(D-α-Sulfoaminophenyl-acetamido) penicillin	Pivaloyloxymethyl ester	Oral	Absorption	26

TABLE III. (Continued)

Parent Molecule	Chemical Modification	Route of Administration	Property Modified	Reference
8. Hetacillin	Pivaloyloxymethyl ester	Oral	Absorption	6
9. Carbenicillin	a. Mono and bis alkyl esters	Oral	Absorption	10
	b. Indanyl ester	Oral	Absorption	9,12
	c. Thienyl esters	Oral	Absorption	27
10. 6-(3-Thienyloxyacetamido) penicillin	Acetoxymethyl ester	Oral	Absorption, duration of activity	31
11. Acetamidopenicillins	Carboxamido ester	IM	Duration of activity	28
12. α-Aminobenzyl penicillin	Dibenzylethylene diamine salt	IM	Duration of activity	29
13. Pivaloyloxymethyl-D-α-aminobenzylpenicillinate	Probenecid salt	Oral	Bitterness	30
14. Penicillin, general structure	a. Chalcon-4-yl esters	Oral	Resistance to penicillinase	33
	b. Amide	Oral	Resistance to penicillinase	34

An alternative procedure (Scheme XI) involves deacetylation of the potassium salt of 25 with citrus acetyl esterase (orange peel enzyme) to afford potassium 7-(2'-thienylacetamido) cephalospora-desate[1] 30 in good yield without isomerization to the Δ^2 derivative (45,46). Acylation of the 3-hydroxymethyl group is base dependent. Conventional attempts at acylation under acidic conditions, e.g. acetic anhydride, produce cephalosporadesolactones. Aromatic ester derivatives are made, however, by employing the conditions of the Schotten-Baumann reaction. Thus, treatment of 30 with a large excess of benzoyl chloride and sodium hydroxide in aqueous acetone affords a good yield of sodium O-benzoyl-7-(2'-thienylacetamido) cephalosporadesate 31. Aliphatic acid chlorides under the same conditions react preferentially with water and no esterification occurs.

C₄ esters. The cephalosporin C_4 esters are synthesized by conventional methods (47). (Scheme XII). Addition of equi-molar quantities of triethylamine (TEA) and isobutyl chlorofor-mate to 25 gave 7-(2'-thienylacetamido) cephalosporanic acid mono-isobutylcarbonate anhydride 32 as an oil which was subsequently obtained crystalline. The ethylcarbonate anhydride was also prepared by this method. Further attempts to esterify at C_4 via the mixed anhydride resulted in mixtures of Δ^2 and Δ^3 esters. Efforts to separate the isomeric esters by recrystallization were unsuccessful.

C₄ amides. Two approaches have been utilized in an effort to form cephalosporin C_4 amides. The first involves the direct condensation of cephalothin with N,N'-dicyclohexylcarbodiimide (DCC) to form the activated carboxyl intermediate. (Scheme XIII). The exchange reaction with t-butyl-α-aminopropionate to form N-{1-carbo-t-butoxy)ethyl}-7-(2'-thienylacetamido) cephalospor-anic acid amide 33 proceeds without isomerization. The alterna-tive approach is somewhat more involved and provides the C_4 amide as the Δ^2 isomer. (Scheme XIV) (47). The procedure of Nefkens et.al. (48) was followed to produce the activated car-bonyl intermediate. Thus, 25, N-hydroxyphthalimide (phthaloxime, 34) and DCC were stirred together and stored for several days. Work up of the reaction mixture gave a 50% yield of N-{7-(2'-thienylacetamido) cephalosporanoyloxy} phthalimide 35. The reac-tion of 35 with ethyl glycinate afforded a 73% yield of completely isomerized Δ^2 amide, N-(carbethoxymethyl)-3-acetoxymethyl-7-(2'-thienylacetamido)-2-cephem-4-carboxylic acid amide 36. Other

_____

[1]Desacetylcephalosporins have been trivially named cephalos-poradesic acids for convenience.

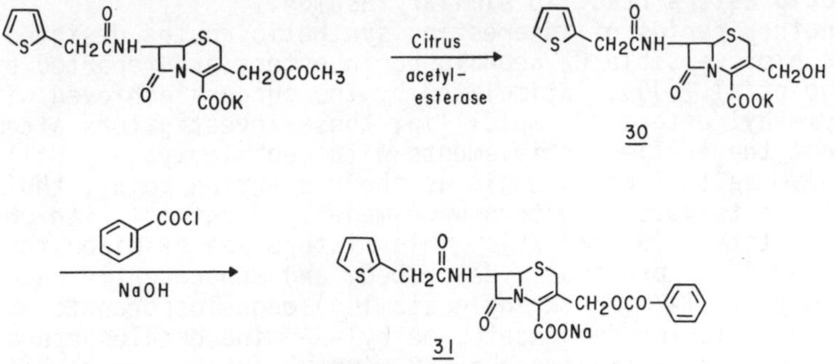

Scheme XI

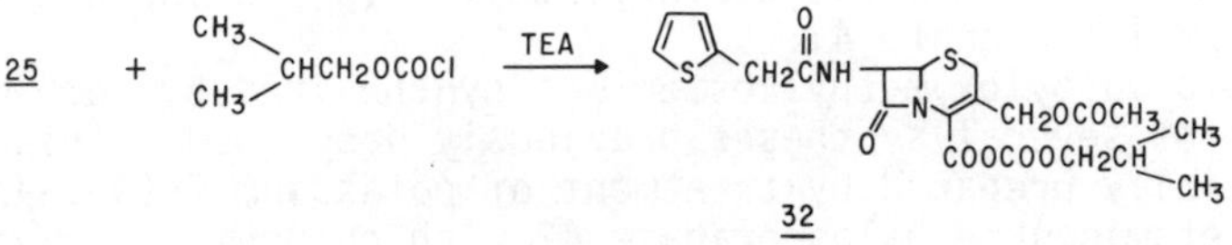

Scheme XII

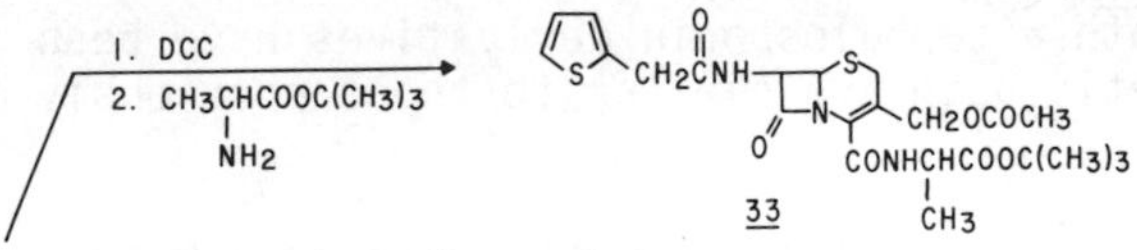

Scheme XIII

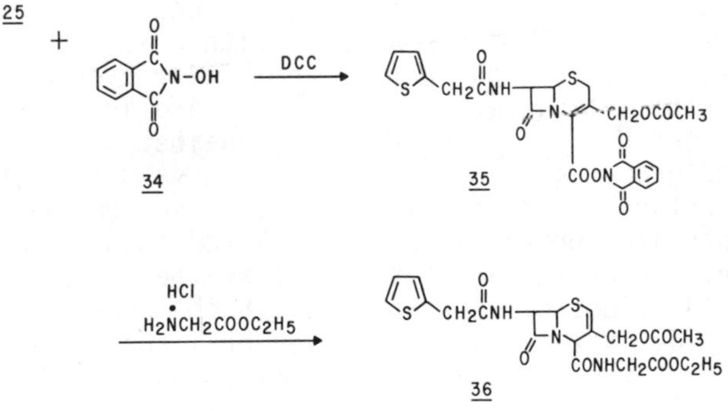

Scheme XIV

amino acid esters react in similar fashion.

Another series of interesting synthetic routes designed to provide bioreversible C_4 cephalosporin esters are reported by Binderup et.al. (49). Stimulated by the success achieved with acyloxymethyl esters of ampicillin, these investigators attempted to repeat the earlier achievements with cephaloglycin. Utilizing the sodium salt of cephalothin as their starting point, the Δ^2 and Δ^3 acetoxymethyl esters were made by treatment with chloro-methyl acetate. (Scheme XV). This mixture was oxidized to the sulfoxide 37, as previously described, and subsequently reduced to acetoxymethyl-7-(2'-thienylacetamido) cephalosporanate 38 with phosphorus trichloride. Acetoxymethyl-7-aminocephalosporanate 39 was produced by treatment of 38 with phosphorus pentachloride and n-propanol. The hydrochloride salt of 39 was formed by the addition of 1N HCl. To 39 was added D-α-azidophenylacetyl chloride to yield acetoxymethyl-7-(D-α-azidophenylacetamido) cephalosporanate 40 which was subsequently hydrogenated with 10% palladium/carbon to yield acetoxymethyl-7-(D-α-aminophenylaceta-mido) cephalosporanate 41.

The pivaloyloxymethyl ester was synthesized by combining features of several syntheses previously described. This ester was initially prepared by treatment of potassium 7-(D-α-azido-phenylacetamido) cephalosporanate 42 with chloromethylpivalate. A mixture of the Δ^2 43 and Δ^3 esters were formed by this proce-dure. Treatment of the mixture first with m-chloroperbenzoic acid to form the sulfoxide Δ^3 ester and secondly with sodium dithionite/acetyl chloride gave the requisite pivaloyloxymethyl-7-(D-α-azidophenylacetamido) cephalosporanate 44 exclusively as the Δ^3 isomer. Reduction of 44 by catalytic hydrogenation af-forded pivaloyloxymethyl-7-(D-α-aminophenylacetamido) cephalo-sporanate 45.

Many other cephalosporin derivatives have been made utili-zing synthetic pathways similar to those previously discussed (50-53).

Biological. Several attempts have been made to improve certain physicochemical and biological properties (especially GI absorption) of the cephalosporins by the prodrug approach. Most efforts have been only moderately successful. Kukolja (44) replaced the 3-acetate of cephalothin with a series of sterically hindered esters for the purpose of inhibiting hydrolysis at this position on the antibiotic. The butyrate and isobutyrate deriva-tives exhibited good in vitro activity against a variety of gram-positive and gram-negative bacteria. ED_{50} values in mice in-dicated bioactivity somewhat improved over sodium cephalothin. The cyclobutyrate derivative also exhibited good broad-spectrum bioactivity. Chauvette and Flynn (47) synthesized a variety of C_4 esters and amides of cephalothin with the specific objective of obtaining derivatives with improved oral absorption. On ad-ministration of these derivatives to mice, a low order of antibacterial activity was found (as measured by levels of antibiotic in the blood).

A series of C_3 aroyl derivatives of cephalothin and 7-phenyl-mercaptoacetamidocephalosporanic acid were made by Van Heyningen (46) and found to possess no significantly improved bioactivity over the parent antibiotics.

The synthetic and bioactivity studies of Binderup et.al. (49) with the acyloxymethyl esters of cephaloglycin represent the first major success in obtaining a superior orally absorbed pro-drug of a cephalosporin. The synthesis of the C_4 acetoxymethyl ester 41 and the pivaloyloxymethyl ester of cephaloglycin 45 are detailed in Scheme XVI. The half-lives of 41 and 45 in 10% human serum are 5 minutes and 10-20 minutes respectively. The absorption and excretion patterns of these derivatives in man (cross-over study in four fasting, healthy volunteers) indicate efficient absorption and rapid ester hydrolysis after absorption. Figure 1 illustrates serum levels obtained with these esters vs. cephaloglycin. Recovery of cephaloglycin in the urine during six hours after administration represented 68% (acetoxymethyl ester) and 61% (pivaloyloxymethyl ester) of the theoretical amount administered. The corresponding average figure for cephaloglycin was 18%.

Cephalosporins viewed as prodrugs. When administered to animals and man, several of the cephalosporins are metabolized to the correspondingly bioactive desacetyl cephalosporin. These C_3 acyloxymethyl esters can, therefore, be considered cephalosporin prodrugs, e.g., cephalothin is enzymatically and/or chemically hydrolyzed in vivo to the bioactive desacetylcephalothin (54,55). Further, the lactones of certain desacetyl cephalosporins exhibit activity against a strain of Staphylococcus aureus that is equal to that of the parent cephalosporin (56), indicating that perhaps the lactone may also be considered a cephalosporin prodrug.

Studies on the metabolic fate of cephaloglycin in the rat by Sullivan and coworkers (57) have demonstrated that a large amount of the oral absorbed dose of this antibiotic is excreted as desacetylcephaloglycin. Approximately 70% of the administered dose is recovered in the feces indicating poor GI absorption. Parenterally administered cephaloglycin is also metabolized primarily to desacetylcephaloglycin. In the mouse, Wick, et.al. (58) found orally administered cephaloglycin in urine in a 1:1 ratio with desacetylcephaloglycin. The principal metabolite of cephaloglycin in humans is desacetylcephaloglycin and is equivalent in activity against gram-positive organisms but is less active against gram-negative organisms. Eradication of urinary tract infections is attributed mainly to the bioactivity of the desacetyl derivative suggesting that cephaloglycin may be the prodrug derivative of desacetylcephaloglycin.

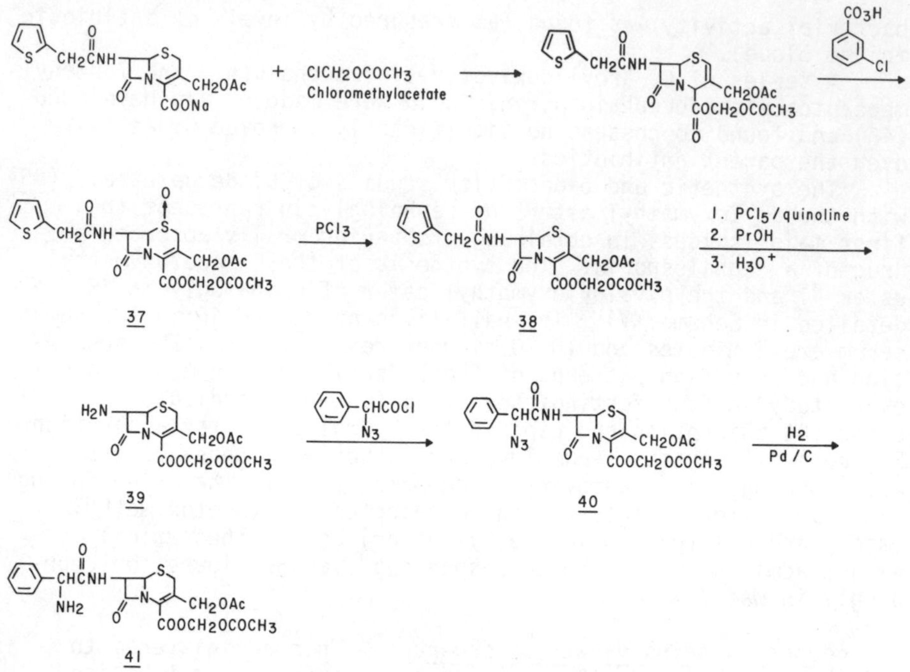
ClCH2OCOCH3
Chloromethylacetate
CO3H
Cl
PCl3
1. PCl5 / quinoline
2. PrOH
3. H3O+
37
38
39
40
41
H2
Pd / C

Scheme XV

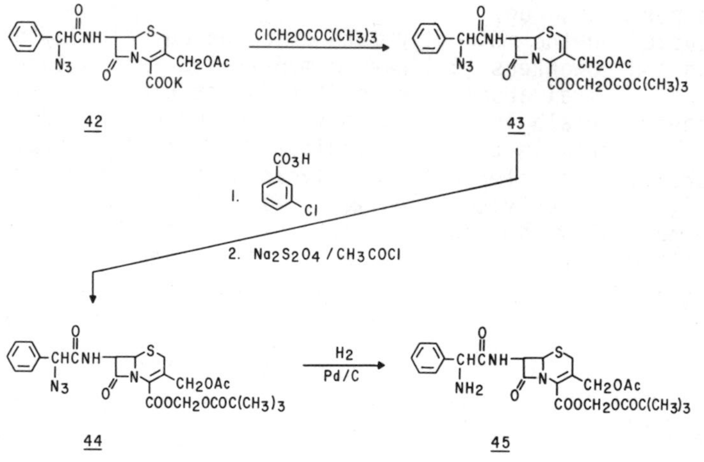
ClCH2OCOC(CH3)3
42
43
CO3H
1.
Cl
2. Na2S2O4 / CH3COCl
H2
Pd/C
44
45

Scheme XVI

Table IV contains several additional cephalosporin prodrugs designed for a variety of uses in medical practice.

Rifampicin

The rifamycins, a family of antibiotics isolated from the fermentation broth of Streptomyces mediterranei n. sp., are currently used in clinical practice against gram-positive microorganisms and tubercular infections (mycobacteria). Of several rifamycins, rifamycin SV and rifamycin B diethylamide are used parenterally against these bacterial infections. Rifamycin SV, moreover, achieves extremely high bile concentrations and is used in infections of the biliary tract. The availability of 3-formyl rifamycin SV 46 led to the synthesis of a large number of rifamycin derivatives designed to provide an orally absorbed form of this antibiotic (70-72). One derivative, {3-(4-methyl-piperazinyliminomethyl) rifamycin SV}, 47, (rifampicin) protects mice against experimental staphylococcal infections at low oral doses (≈0.1 mg./kg.). In man, it is of low toxicity and well absorbed orally (73-75). While elimination occurs mainly through the bile (enterohepatic circulation), small amounts are also found in urine. Thin layer chromatography studies indicated that 47 was almost entirely converted to desacetylrifampicin 48 in vivo and was probably the active antibacterial form of this antibiotic. Thus, while irreversible modification of 3-formyl rifamycin SV to rifampicin enhances oral absorption, in vivo deacetylation of the C_{25} acetate liberates 48, the true parent bioactive species of this antibiotic. (Scheme XVII). Rifampicin, then, represents the prodrug form of desacetylrifampicin. This fact is corroborated by antibacterial studies with desacetyl-rifampicin in man in which the bioactivity is found to be excellent against gram-positive bacteria (76). Oral administration of a 150 mg. dose of rifampicin in man produces bile levels of desacetylrifampicin in excess of 95% over a 5 hour period. No other metabolites are present (77).

Clindamycin

Clindamycin {7(S)-chloro-7-deoxylincomycin} hydrochloride 49 is a semisynthetic antibiotic derived from lincomycin. Its activity against gram-positive aerobes and gram-positive and gram-negative anaerobic pathogens is greater than that of lincomycin. Clindamycin is well absorbed from the GI tract and produces serum levels considerably greater than lincomycin (78-80). The extreme bitterness of clindamycin precludes its solution or suspension formulation as an acceptable oral dosage form. Further, the incidence of pain at the injection site after intramuscular injection is considerable. These undesirable properties of clindamycin prompted a search for prodrug derivatives of this antibiotic designed to enhance its acceptability.

TABLE IV. CEPHALOSPORIN PRODRUGS DESIGNED TO MODIFY VARIOUS PROPERTIES OF THE PARENT ANTIBIOTIC

Parent Molecule	Chemical Modification	Route of Administration	Property Modified	Reference
1. 7-Acylcephalosporanic Acid	a. C_4-alkoxycarbonyloxy-alkyl esters	Oral	Absorption	59
	b. C_4-aryloxycarbonyloxy-alkyl esters			
	c. C_4-alkoxycarbonylamino-alkyl esters			
2. 7-Acylaminocephalosporanic acid	C_4-p-alkoxycarbonyloxybenzyl esters	Oral	Absorption	60
3. 7-Acylaminocephalosporanic acid	C_4-acyloxyalkyl esters	Oral	Absorption, decreased toxicity	61
4. 7-Acylaminodesacetoxy cephalosporanic acid	C_4-acyloxybenzyl esters	Oral	Absorption	62
5. 7-Acylcephalosporanic acid	C_3-benzhydryl esters	Oral	Absorption	63

TABLE IV.   (Continued)

	Parent Molecule	Chemical Modification	Route of Administration	Property Modified	Reference
6.	7-Acylaminocephalosporanic acid	Imino ether	Oral	Decreased toxicity, resistance to β-lactamase	64
7.	7-α-Amino (or ureido) cyclo-hexadienylalkyl cephalosporanic acid	C$_4$-acyloxymethyl esters	Oral	Absorption	65
8.	7-Substituted cephalosporanic acid	C$_4$-Aminoacyloxymethyl esters	Oral	Absorption, increased water solubility, decreased side effects	66
9.	Substituted 7-β-aminocephem-4-carboxylic acid	C$_4$-physiologically labile esters	Oral	Absorption	67-69

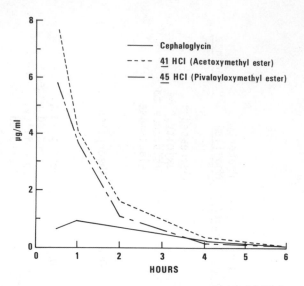

Journal of Antibiotics

Figure 1. Mean serum levels of cephaloglycin in fasting, healthy volunteers following oral administration of 200 mg of cephaloglycin and equimolar amounts of 41 HCl and 45 HCl (49)

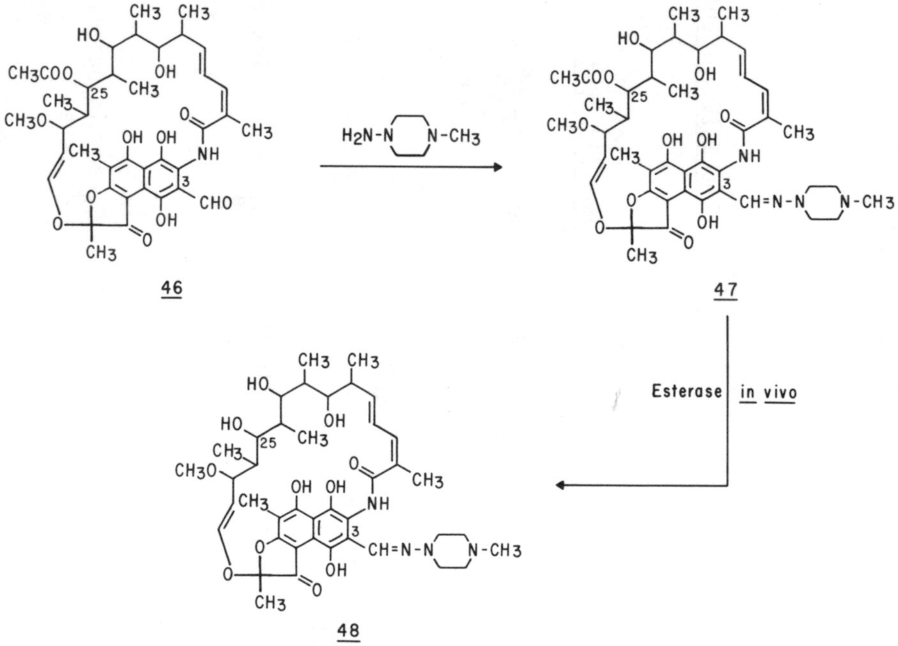

Scheme XVII

For prodrug purposes, clindamycin can be chemically modified
at any of the three hydroxyl groups present on the sugar portion
of the molecule.

Clindamycin Alkyl Esters. Biologically reversible alkyl
esters were sought that would eliminate the bitter taste of
clindamycin by decreasing aqueous solubility below taste threshold
levels.

Chemistry. Standard synthetic procedures were utilized in
the synthesis of 2- and 3-monoesters and 2,3-bis alkyl esters.
(Schemes XVIII - XX). (81).
Clindamycin-2-esters are synthesized by utilizing 3,4-O-p-
anisylidene-7(S)-chloro-7-deoxylincomycin 50 in which the 3 and
4 hydroxyl groups are blocked by an acetal. The C_2 hydroxyl
is esterified with either an alkyl anhydride, an acid chloride
or an alkyl chloroformate and the ester-acetal hydrolyzed in
acidic media to the 2-acyl ester of clindamycin.
Selective esterification of the 3 hydroxyl group is achieved
by the use of a low temperature reaction medium (pyridine at -25°
C) and a two-fold excess of alkyl chloroformate.
The 2,3-bis esters are made by treatment of 49 with excess
acylating agent and using to advantage the stereochemistry of
the hydroxyl groups. The C_2 and C_3 hydroxyl groups are equatorial
and relatively chemically reactive whereas the C_4 hydroxyl is
axial and is not esterified to any appreciable extent under these
conditions.

In vitro and in vivo studies. Table V lists preliminary
antibacterial activities of selected clindamycin esters using the
mouse as the model test system (81). In vitro data for all ester
derivatives show activity less than clindamycin. This appears
reasonable since many other esterified antibiotics have been
shown to be inactive until hydrolysis occurs (82-83).
The in vivo CD_{50} data in mice indicate that virtually none
of the esters possess activity comparable to clindamycin. Subsequent blood level studies in dogs, however, provided ample
evidence that several 2-acyl esters were equivalent in activity
(as measured by serum concentration of clindamycin released from
ester) to clindamycin HCl (81). This difference in bioactivity
between two animal species illustrates the importance of testing
prodrug antibiotics in several species before a decision is
made to eliminate a potential candidate from further testing
in other animal species or in man.
Clindamycin-2-palmitate and -2-hexadecylcarbonate were
selected for comparative bioavailability studies because (1)
following oral administration to dogs, each ester produced serum
clindamycin levels equivalent to those obtained with clindamycin
HCl and (2) the esters lacked the characteristic bitterness of
clindamycin.

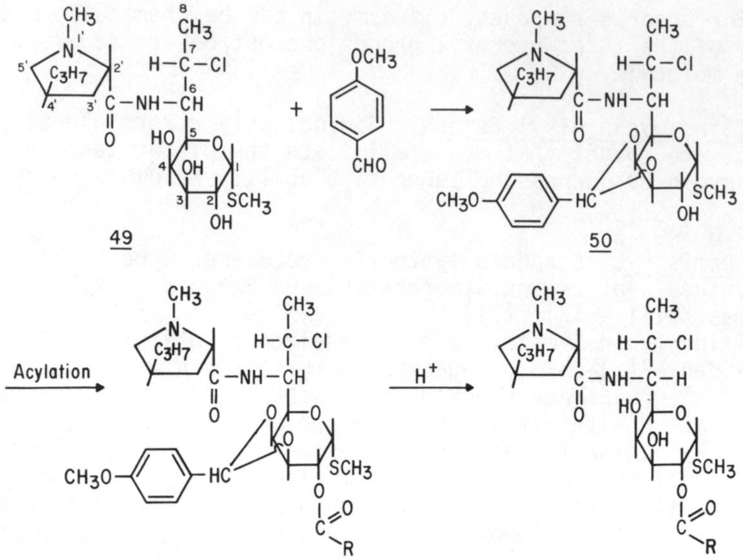

Scheme XVIII.   Clindamycin-2-monoesters

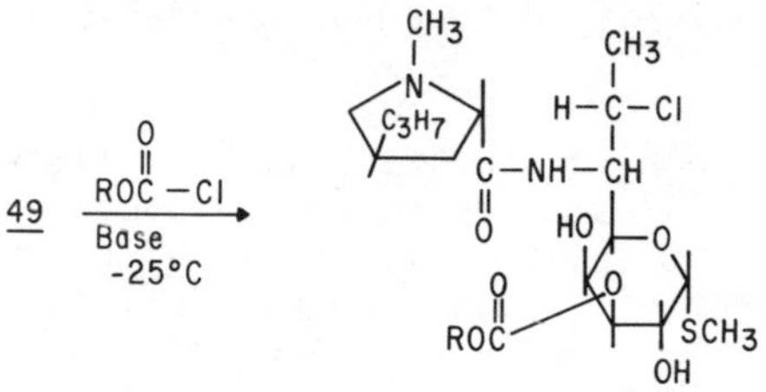

Scheme XIX.   Clindamycin-3-monocarbonate esters

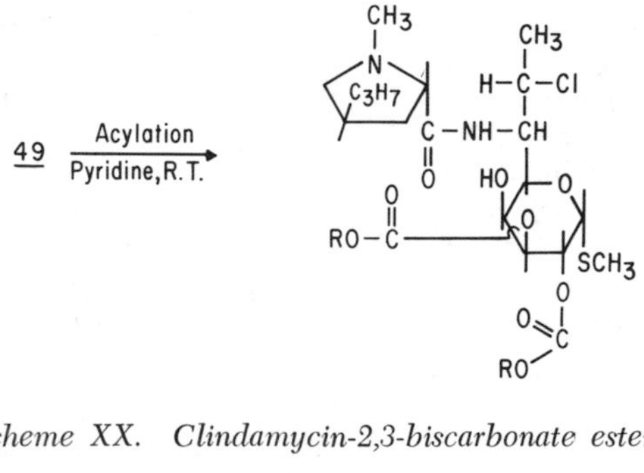

Scheme XX.   Clindamycin-2,3-biscarbonate esters

TABLE V. ANTIBACTERIAL ACTIVITY OF CLINDAMYCIN 2- and 3-MONOESTERS AND 2,3-DIESTERS[a]

	In Vitro Activity[b] mcg./mg.	Antibacterial Activity Relative Median Protective Dose (CD_{50})[c]	
		Subcutaneous	Oral
Clindamycin 2-hexanoate hydrochloride	690 (69)	1.31	0.67
Clindamycin 2-hexylcarbonate hydrochloride	330 (33)	1.36	0.43
Clindamycin 2-laurate hydrochloride	20 (2.0)	<0.1	<0.28
Clindamycin 2-palmitate hydrochloride	21 (2.1)	<0.3	0.21
Clindamycin 2-hexadecylcarbonate hydrochloride	<4 (<0.4)	<0.1	0.23
Clindamycin 2-(p-benzoyl) benzoate hydrochloride	55 (5.5)	1.67	0.54
Clindamycin 2-(o-benzoyl) benzoate hydrochloride	7 (0.7)	<0.15	0.29
Clindamycin 3-pentylcarbonate hydrochloride	180 (18)	0.37	0.67
Clindamycin 2,3-bis (hexylcarbonate) hydrochloride	<4 (<0.4)	0.18	0.60

[a]Activities calculated as clindamycin base equivalents. [b]As measured on a standard curve agar assay versus <u>Sarcina lutea</u>. Results expressed as micrograms of clindamycin base activity per milligram of ester and as percent of lincomycin base activity (in parenthesis). [c]Median protective dose relative to that of clindamycin (clindamycin = 1.0) in the mouse. (81).

JOURNAL OF PHARMACEUTICAL SCIENCES

Following a study of the two esters and clindamycin HCl in twelve healthy male volunteers, Forist et.al. (84) fitted the resulting serum concentration data to a one-compartment open pharmacokinetic model.

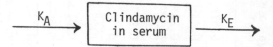

K_A represents the first-order rate constant for appearance of clindamycin in the serum. Both hydrolysis and absorption are represented in this constant for the esters. K_E represents the first-order rate constant for elimination of clindamycin from the body. Other parameters calculated by treatment of this data included half-lives for appearance ($A_{\frac{1}{2}}$) and elimination ($E_{\frac{1}{2}}$) of bioactivity, serum concentration maximum and time of maximum concentration as well as area under the concentration vs. time curve ($0 \longrightarrow \infty$) and are listed in Table VI.

The rate of appearance ($A_{\frac{1}{2}}$) of clindamycin and the palmitate ester in serum are not significantly different from each other but both were more rapidly absorbed than the hexadecylcarbonate ester. It appears that clindamycin-2-hexadecylcarbonate may not be hydrolyzed as rapidly or as completely as the palmitate ester. This observation is further substantiated by a comparison of the serum concentration maxima, the estimated time of maximum concentration and total area under the concentration vs. time curve for the two esters. Based on this study, clindamycin-2-palmitate became the candidate of choice for further clinical trials. Subsequent investigations on larger patient populations have verified the results of this twelve subject study (85-89).

Clindamycin-2-phosphate. The phosphate ester of clindamycin was synthesized to provide a bioreversible form of clindamycin devoid of pain and irritation upon injection. The irritation caused by injectable clindamycin was thought to arise from precipitation of the free base at the site of injection or lysis due to drug partitioning into cells surrounding the injection site. At physiological pH (7.4) clindamycin HCl is soluble only to the extent of 3 mg./ml. whereas clindamycin-2-phosphate is readily soluble at this pH (>150 mg./ml.) and should not precipitate at the injection site. Further, penetration of clindamycin-2-phosphate into the cell should be negligible since its lipophilic character is drastically diminished via the hydrophilic phosphate ester.

Chemistry (90,91). The C_3 and C_4 hydroxyl groups of clindamycin are chemically blocked by formation of 3,4-O-p-anisylidene-7(S)-chloro-7-deoxylincomycin 50. (Scheme XXI). Treatment of 50 with cyanoethyl phosphate and dicyclohexylcarbodiimide (DCC)

<u>TABLE VI</u>

Pharmacokinetic Parameters Estimated from Serum Clindamycin Bioactivity Concentrations Following Oral Administration (150 mg.)
of Clindamycin-2-Palmitate (A), Clindamycin-2-Hexadecylcarbonate
(B), and Clindamycin Hydrochloride (C)

Parameter	A	B	C
K_A (hr.$^{-1}$)	2.81(0.92)[a]	1.53(0.94)	7.65(7.56)
	1.23-4.38[b]	0.75-3.41	1.03-22.92
	2.75[c]	0.92	4.66
$A_{\frac{1}{2}}$ (hr.)	0.28(0.11)	0.58(0.25)	0.19(0.18)
	0.16-0.56	0.20-0.93	0.03-0.67
	0.25	0.76	0.15
Estimated time of maximum concentration (hr.)	1.16(0.24)	1.67(0.32)	0.86(0.53)
	0.86-1.62	1.09-2.09	0.19-1.88
	1.15	1.80	0.78
Estimated maximum concentration (μg/ml)	1.99(0.61)	1.47(0.48)	2.61(1.14)
	1.29-3.34	0.97-2.33	1.75-5.75
	1.97	1.44	2.38
Observed maximum concentration (μg/ml)	2.05(0.66)	1.47(0.54)	2.80(1.26)
	1.33-3.38	0.96-2.39	1.67-6.40
	2.05	1.42	2.39
K_E (hr.$^{-1}$)	0.25(0.07)	0.35(0.19)	0.26(0.07)
	0.17-0.35	0.17-0.81	0.18-0.35
	0.24	0.36	0.23
$E_{\frac{1}{2}}$ (hr.)	2.94(0.83)	2.48(1.14)	2.84(0.76)
	2.00-4.08	0.85-4.17	2.00-3.93
	2.83	1.95	3.04
Area, $0 \longrightarrow \infty$ (μg hr./ml)	10.68(4.04)	8.22(3.85)	12.33(4.37)
	5.63-21.14	3.71-15.40	8.36-20.04
	10.20	7.37	12.20

JOURNAL OF PHARMACOKINETICS AND BIOPHARMACEUTICS

[a]Mean (SD) for 12 subjects.
[b]Range.
[c]Average obtained from mean serum levels for 12 subjects. (<u>84</u>).

yields the cyanoethyl phosphate ester intermediate 51 which is converted to clindamycin-2-cyanoethyl phosphate 52 after acid treatment. The intermediate 51 is purified by recrystallization from water. Base hydrolysis of the phosphodiester with ammonium hydroxide on a TEAE-cellulose column packed with 1N ammonium acetate affords clindamycin-2-phosphate 53.

An alternative procedure involves the treatment of 50 with POCl$_3$/pyridine. Addition of water yields the phosphomonoester 3,4-0-anisylidene acetal 54. Acid hydrolysis of the acetal leads to good yields of 53.

Bioactivity. Clindamycin-2-phosphate activity in vitro is very low (<1%) indicating that the phosphate ester possesses very little, if any, antibacterial activity per se (92). The median protective dose (CD$_{50}$) of clindamycin-2-phosphate in mice infected with Staphylococcus aureus is somewhat higher than for clindamycin HCl (6.6 mg./kg. vs. 4.9 mg./kg.), reflecting a slowed rate of hydrolysis of the bioinactive ester. Single subcutaneous doses of 10 mg./kg. in rats produce lower blood levels for the phosphate vs. clindamycin again indicating that the phosphate ester experiences a slight delay in hydrolysis in vivo. This study is summarized in Table VII (92).

Clinical studies in human volunteers reveal a pattern similar to that found in the lower animal species. Thus, DeHaan et.al., (93) found that the ester is absorbed intact after multiple intramuscular injections but is rapidly hydrolyzed in the serum (Figure 2). In fact, after a ten minute intravenous infusion of clindamycin phosphate, the mean half-life of the ester in serum is estimated to be 9.6 minutes (Figure 3) verifying the rapid conversion of bioinactive ester to clindamycin.

Other studies in animals (94) and in man (95) have demonstrated the lack of local irritation and pain with injectable clindamycin phosphate.

Summary

This brief review highlights the importance of the use of an interdisciplinary approach in the synthesis and testing of antibiotic prodrug derivatives. Along with the development of unique chemistry for the synthesis of such prodrugs, a knowledge and appreciation of the various in vitro and in vivo methods of biological evaluation of such derivatives is necessary to rationally choose those best suited for clinical use. Further, selected pharmacokinetic studies are valuable in the determination of the absorption, distribution, metabolism, and elimination characteristics of such drugs.

TABLE VII

Comparative bioactivities in whole blood of rats after a single subcutaneous dose of clindamycin and clindamycin 2-PO_4 at 10 mg./kg.[a].

Antibiotic	Area under curve ± 2 SE[b]	Relative area of curves[c]	Mean time of 50% area ± 2 SE[d]	Max. conc. (mcg/ml) at time *t*
Clindamycin	177 ± 30	1.00	72 ± 10	2.25 mcg/ml at 30 min
Clindamycin-2-PO_4	136 ± 32	0.76	74 ± 5	1.23 mcg/ml at 45 min

JOURNAL OF ANTIBIOTICS

[a] Calculated as molecular equivalents of clindamycin base.

[b] Area under time : concentration curve ± standard errors. Values represent mean of three determinations with 3 rats per determination.

[c] Area values relative to that of clindamycin. Clindamycin = 1.00.

[d] Time (min) at which 50% of area is under the time : concentration curve. (92).

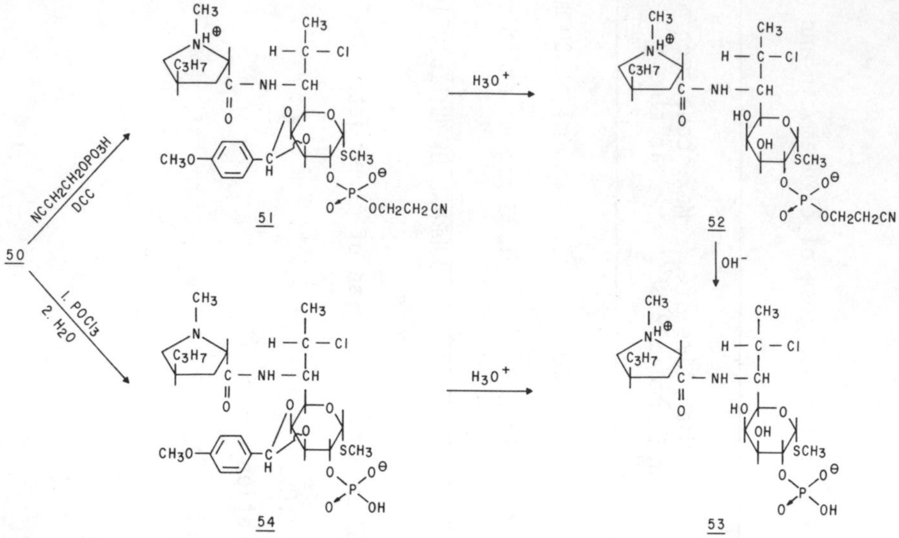

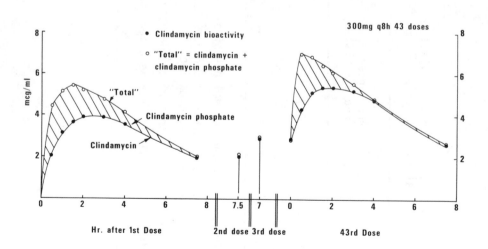

Scheme XXI

Journal of Clinical Pharmacology

Figure 2. Mean serum concentrations (μg/ml) of clindamycin and clindamycin phosphate after I.M. injections of clindamycin phosphate (93)

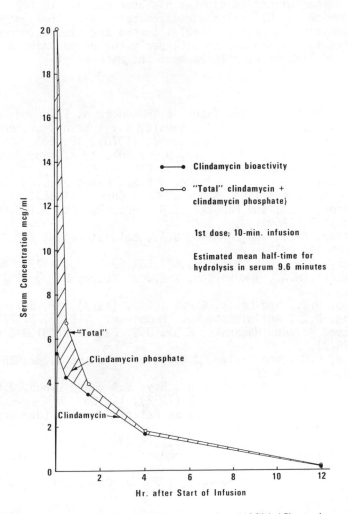

Journal of Clinical Pharmacology

Figure 3.   Mean serum concentrations (μg/ml) of clindamycin and clindamycin phosphate after a 300-mg I.V. infusion of clindamycin phosphate (10-min infusion) (93)

Acknowledgements

The author wishes to express his appreciation to Dr.
W. Morozowich for helpful suggestions concerning the synthesis
of clindamycin phosphate. Special thanks are also extended to
D. Harling for typing and to E.E. Beals for preparation of the
schemes and figures used throughout the manuscript.

Literature Cited

1. von Daehne, W., Frederiksen, E., Gunderson, E., Lund, F.,
    Mørch, P., Petersen, H.J., Roholt, K., Tybring, L., and
    Godtfredsen, W.O., J. Med. Chem., (1970), 13, 607.
2. von Daehne, W., Godtfredsen, W.O., Roholt, K., and Tybring,
    L., Antimicrob. Ag. Chemother., (1970), 431.
3. Hardcastle, G.A., Jr., Johnson, D.A., Panetta, C.A., Scott,
    A.I., and Sutherland, S.A., J. Org. Chem., (1966), 31, 897.
4. Johnson, D.A., and Panetta, C.A., U.S. Patent, 3,198,804
    (August 3, 1965).
5. Sleezer, P.D., and Johnson, D.A., Belgian Patent 788,720
    (March 12, 1973).
6. Essery, J.M., U.S. Patent 3,679,663 (July 25, 1972).
7. Schwartz, M.A., and Hayton, W.L., J. Pharm. Sci., (1972), 61,
    906.
8. Jusko, W.J., and Lewis, G.P., Ibid., (1973), 62, 69.
9. Hobbs, D.C., Antimicrob. Ag. Chemother., (1972), 2, 272.
10. Butler, K., and Hamanaka, E.S., U.S. Patent 3,681,342 (August
    1, 1972).
11. Brain, E.G., and Nayler, J.H.C., U.S. Patent 3,282,926
    (November 1, 1966).
12. English, A.R., Retsema, J.A., Ray, V.A., and Lynch, J.E.,
    Antimicrob. Ag. Chemother., (1972), 1, 185.
13. Farbwerke Hoechst, Netherlands Patent 73,09128 (January 8,
    1974).
14. Petersen, H.J., J. Med. Chem., (1974), 17, 101.
15. Frederiksen, E.K., and Godtfredsen, W.O., U.S. Patent 3,719,
    668 (March 6, 1973).
16. Jensen, A.B.A., and Russell, T.J., J. Chem. Soc., (1965),
    2127.
17. Hansson, E., Magni, L., and Wahlgvist, S., Antimicrob. Ag.
    Chemother., (1967), 568.
18. Ramsey, C.H., Bodin, N.O., and Hansson, E., Arzneim. -Forsch.
    (1972), 22, 1962.
19. Foltz, E.L., West, J.W., Breslow, I.H., and Wallick, H.,
    Antimicrob. Ag. Chemother., (1970), 442.
20. Jordan, M.C., deMaine, J.B., and Kirby, W.M.M., Ibid., 438.
21. Hultberg, E.R., and Backelin, B., Scand. J. Infect. Dis.,
    (1972), 4, 149.

22. Frederiksen, E.K., and Godtfredsen, W.O., U.S. Patent 3,697, 507 (October 10, 1972).
23. Jusko, W.J., Lewis, G.P., and Schmitt, G.W., Clin. Pharmacol. Ther., (1973), 14, 90.
24. Yurchenco, J.A., Hopper, M.W., Vince, T.D., and Warren, G.H., Chemotherapy, (1972), 17, 405.
25. E.R. Squibb and Sons, Inc., West German Patent 2,152,745 (April 27, 1972).
26. Essery, J.M., and West, J.R., U.S. Patent 3,654,265 (April 4, 1972).
27. Farbwerke Hoechst AG, Netherlands Patent 7,309,129 (January 8, 1974).
28. Sellstedt, J.H., and Wolf, M., U.S. Patent 3,692,774 (September 19, 1972).
29. Andreu, SA, West German Patent 2,237,267 (February 1, 1973).
30. Merck and Co., Inc., West German Patent 2,256,538 (May 24, 1973).
31. Farbwerke Hoechst AG, West German Patent 2,159,555 (June 7, 1973).
32. Beecham Group Ltd., Belgian Patent 784,698 (December 11, 1972).
33. Soc. Rech. et Applic. Ind., French Patent 2,181,505 (December 7, 1973).
34. Soc. Rech. et Applic. Ind., French Patent 2,181,506 (December 7, 1973).
35. Boniece, W.S., Wick, W.E., Holmes, D.H., and Redman, C.E., J. Bacteriol.,(1962), 84, 1292.
36. Naumann, P., and Fedder, J., Int. J. Clin. Pharmacol. Beiheft Oracef., (1970), 6.
37. Wick, W.E., in "Cephalosporins and Penicillins - Chemistry and Biology", E.H. Flynn, ed., pp. 515-517, Academic Press, New York, NY, 1972.
38. Wick, W.E., and Boniece, W.S., Appl. Microbiol., (1965), 13, 243.
39. Wick, W.E., Ibid., (1967), 15, 765.
40. Applestein, J.M., Crosby, E.B., Johnson, W.D., and Kaye, D., Ibid., (1968), 16, 1006.
41. Thornhill, T.S., Levison, M.E., Johnson, W.D., and Kaye, D., Ibid., (1969), 17, 457.
42. Flynn, E.H., U.S. Patent 3,218,318 (November 16, 1965).
43. Kukolja, S., U.S. Patent 3,728,342 (April 17, 1973).
44. Kukolja, S., J. Med. Chem., (1970), 13, 1114.
45. Jensen, E.F., Jang, R., and MacDonnell, L.R., Arch. Biochem., (1947), 15, 415.
46. Van Heyningen, E., J. Med. Chem., (1965), 8, 22.
47. Chauvette, R.R., and Flynn, E.H., J. Med. Chem., (1966), 9, 741.
48. Nefkens, G.H.L., Tesser, G.I., and Nivard, R.J.F., Rec. Trav. Chim., (1962), 81, 683.

49. Binderup, E., Godtfredsen, W.O., and Roholt, K., J. Antibiot. (1971), 24, 767.

50. Cheney, L.C., Godfrey, J.C., Crast, L.B., Jr., and Luttinger, J.R., U.S. Patent 3,284,451 (November 6, 1966).

51. Webber, J.A., Huffman, G.W., Koehler, R.E., Murphy, C.F., Ryan, C.W., Van Heyningen, E.M., and Vasileff, R.T., J. Med. Chem., (1971), 14, 113.

52. Jen, T., Dienel, B., Frazee, J., and Weisbach, J., J. Med. Chem., (1972), 15, 1172.

53. Webber, J.A., and Van Heyningen, E.M., U.S. Patent 3,708, 480 (January 2, 1973).

54. Wick, W.E., Antimicrob. Ag. Chemother., (1966), 870.

55. Lee, C.C., Herr, E.B., and Anderson, R.C., Clin. Med., (1963) 70, 1123.

56. Chauvette, R.R., Flynn, E.H., Jackson, B.G., Lavagnino, E.R., Morin, R.B., Mueller, R.A., Pioch, R.P., Roeske, R.W., Ryan, C.W., Spencer, J.L., and Van Heyningen, E., Antimicrob. Ag. Chemother., (1963), 687.

57. Sullivan, H.R., Billings, R.E., and McMahon, R.E., J. Antibiot., (1969), 22, 27.

58. Wick, W.E., Wright, W.E., and Kuder, H.V., Appl. Microbiol., (1971), 21, 426.

59. Astra Lakemedel AB, Netherlands Patent 73,03437 (September 17, 1973).

60. Yamanouchi Pharmaceutical Co. Ltd., Japanese Patent 4,720, 187 (September 27, 1972).

61. Yamanouchi Pharmaceutical Co. Ltd., Belgian Patent 781,659 (July 31, 1972).

62. Yamanouchi Pharmaceutical Co. Ltd., West German Patent 2,223, 588 (August 9, 1973).

63. Merck and Co., Inc., Netherlands Patent 73,09893 (February 5, 1974).

64. Glaxo Labs, Ltd., West German Patent 2,223,375 (November 23, 1972).

65. E.R. Squibb and Sons, Inc., West German Patent 2,152,745 (April 27, 1972).

66. Loevens Kemiske Fab Produktions A/S, West German Patent 2,230,620 (December 28, 1972).

67. Ciba-Geigy AG, Netherlands Patent 73,09136 (January 2, 1974).

68. Ciba-Geigy AG, Netherlands Patent 73,09137 (January 2, 1974).

69. Ciba-Geigy AG, Netherlands Patent 73,09139 (January 2, 1974).

70. Maggi, N., Gallo, G.G., and Sensi, P., Farmaco. Ed. Sci., (1967), 22, 316.

71. Maggi, N., Pallanza, R., and Sensi, P., Antimicrob. Ag. Chemother., (1965), 765.

72. Furesz, S., Arioli, V., and Pallanza, R., Ibid., (1965), 770.

73. Sensi, P.,Maggi, N., Furesz, S., and Maffii, G., Ibid., (1966), 699.

74. Furesz, S., Scotti, R., Pallanza, R., and Mapelli, E., Arzneim. -Forsch., (1967), 17, 726.
75. Acocella, G., Nicolis, F.B., and Lamarina, A., "A Study on the Kinetics of Rifampicin in Man", Vth International Congress of Chemotherapy, Vienna, 1967.
76. Maggi, N., Vigevani, A., and Pallanza, R., Experientia, (1968), 24, 209.
77. Maggi, N., Furesz, S., Pallanza, R., and Pelizza, G., Arzneim.-Forsch, (1969), 19, 651.
78. Wagner, J.G., Novak, E., Patel, N.C. Chidester, C.G., and Lummis, W.L., Amer. J. Med. Sci., (1968), 256, 25.
79. McGehee, R.F., Jr., Smith, C.B., Wilcox, C., and Finland, M., Ibid., 279.
80. DeHaan, R.M., Metzler, C.M., Schellenberg, D., VandenBosch, W.D., and Masson, E.L., Int. J. Clin. Pharmacol., Ther. Toxicol., (1972), 6, 105.
81. Sinkula, A.A., Morozowich, W., and Rowe, E.L., J. Pharm. Sci. (1973), 62, 1106.
82. Wick, W.E., and Mallett, G.E., Antimicrob. Ag. Chemother., (1968), 410.
83. Tardrew, P.L., Mao, J.C.H., and Kenney, D., Appl. Microbiol., (1969), 58, 2140.
84. Forist, A.A., DeHaan, R.M., and Metzler, C.M., J. Pharmacokinet. and Biopharmaceutics, (1973), 1, 89.
85. DeHaan, R.M., VandenBosch, W.D., and Metzler, C.M., J. Clin. Pharmacol., (1972), 12, 205.
86. DeHaan, R.M., and Schellenberg, D., Ibid., (1972), 12, 74.
87. DeHaan, R.M., Schellenberg, D., VandenBosch, W.D., and Maile, M.H., Curr. Ther. Res., (1972), 14, 81.
88. Pfeifer, R.T., DeHaan, R.M., VandenBosch, W.D., and Schellenberg, D., Clin. Med., (1973), 80, 21.
89. Metzler, C.M., DeHaan, R., Schellenberg, D., and VandenBosch, W.D., J. Pharm. Sci., (1973), 62, 591.
90. Morozowich, W., Lamb, D.J., DeHaan, R.M., and Gray, J.E., Abstracts of Papers, APhA Academy of Pharmaceutical Sciences, Washington, D.C. Meeting, April 1970, p. 63.
91. Morozowich, W., and Lamb, D.J., U.S. Patent 3,487,068 (December 30, 1969).
92. Brodasky, T.F., and Lewis, C., J. Antibiot., (1972), 25, 230.
93. DeHaan, R.M., Metzler, C.M., Schellenberg, D., and VandenBosch, W.D., J. Clin. Pharmacol., (1973), 13, 190.
94. Gray, J.E., Weaver, R.N., Moran, J., and Feenstra, E.S., Toxicol. Appl. Pharmacol., (1974), 27, 308.
95. Edmondson, H.T., Ann. Surg., (1973), 178, 637.

3

The Chemistry of a Novel 5,5-Diphenylhydantoin Pro-drug

V. STELLA, T. HIGUCHI, A. HUSSAIN, and J. TRUELOVE

University of Kansas, Department of Pharmaceutical Chemistry and
INTERx Research Corp., Lawrence, Kans. 66044

Phenytoin or 5,5-diphenylhydantoin (DPH), a widely used anticonvulsant agent used primarily in the treatment of grand mal seizures, has shown erratic absorption and dissolution patterns as well as possible precipitation in the body after intravenous (I.V.) infusions of highly alkaline solutions of its sodium salt (1-6). It was the objective of this work to find a water soluble pro-drug (7,8) form of DPH which would revert to DPH in the body. The aim was to improve both the parenteral and oral bioavailability of DPH.

A number of hydantoins including DPH, mephenytoin or 5-ethyl-3-methyl-5-phenylhydantoin (I), and nitrofurantoin or 1-(5-nitro-2-furfurylindene)aminohydantoin (II) are widely used as drugs. Their uses, however, have been hampered by their low water solubility combined with their weakly acidic nature.

Orally the bioavailability of DPH from capsules has been erratic (1-3). The pK_a of DPH, approximately 8.3 (1,9), allows DPH to be formulated as its mono-sodium salt. Formulations of DPH as the free acid are also available. A report before a congressional investigation committee in 1967 suggested that a brand change of DPH resulted in increased convulsive seizures due to lower bioavailability from the new formulation. Similarly differences between products have been noted by Martin et al. (2) and by Arnold et al. (1). The dependency of DPH blood levels after oral dosing on differences, in the rate of metabolism of DPH, particle size, and various generic and trade name products has recently been discussed by Glazko (10). DPH has an aqueous solubility of between 1-4 mg/100 ml (1) and it appears that this poor aqueous solubility is the major cause of the erratic absorption and dissolution rates (1) of

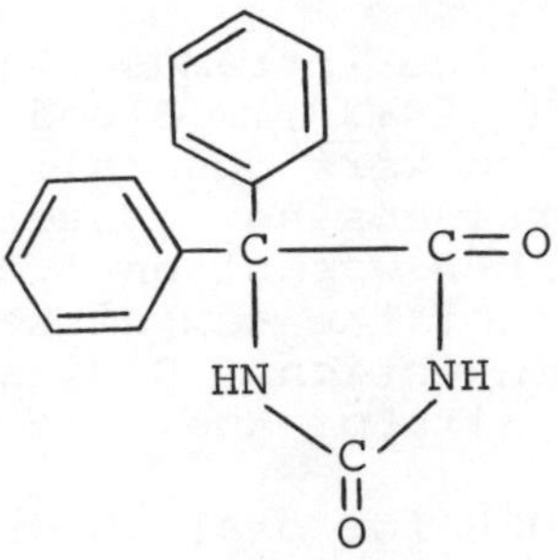

(DPH)

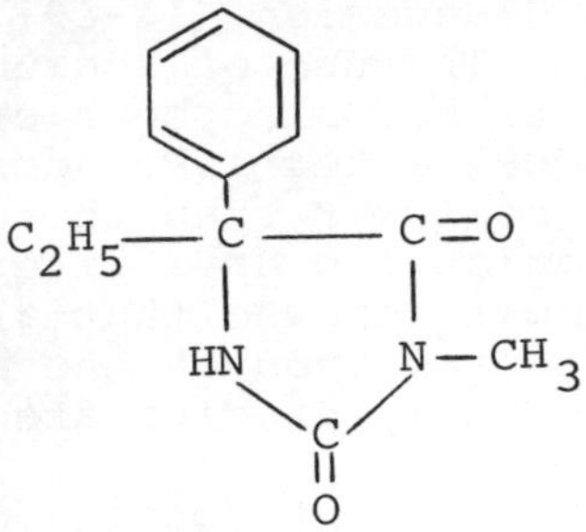

(I)

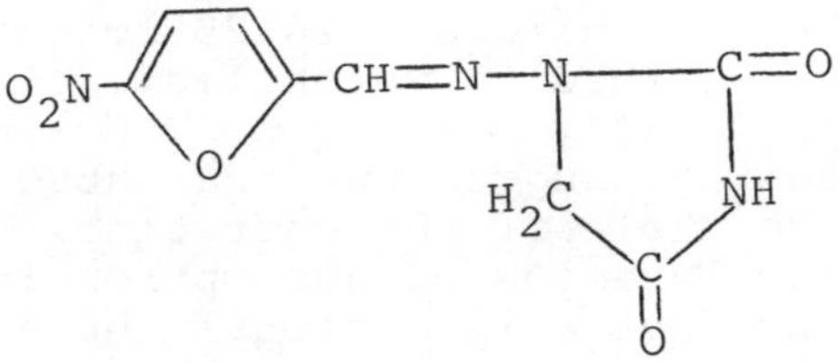

(II)

various DPH preparations. The low aqueous solubility of DPH can be attributed to its strong crystal
lattice (mp. 293) resulting from intermolecular hydrogen bonding (11). That the strong crystal lattice is
a major factor in the determination of solubility is
also exemplified by the poor lipid solubility of DPH.
    DPH is given parenterally as its mono-sodium salt
in a reconstituted injection with a solvent consis-
ting of "40% propylene glycol and 10% alcohol in water
for injection and is buffered to pH 10 to 12 with
sodium hydroxide" (12). Blum et al. (5,6) and others
(13) noted severe side effects in dogs and man when
DPH injections were given intravenously. A subsequent
autopsy of the dogs used in the experiments of Blum
et al. (5,6) showed precipitation of DPH in the lungs,
i.e., the injection of sodium DPH of pH 12 on mixing
with blood buffered at pH 7.4 resulted in the precipitation of DPH as the free acid. Precautions in
the I.V. use of injectable DPH in the treatment of
status epilepticus and digitalis intoxication (13)
and in the attempted preparation of large volume I.V.

injections of DPH have recently been the center
of discussion (14-19).

The use of sodium DPH via the intramuscular (I.M.)
route has also been criticized (20-23). Blood levels
of DPH after I.M. administration were generally found
to be lower than those from oral dosing. Muscle dis-
section two days after sodium DPH was given I.M. to
rabbits showed that almost 50% of the administered
dose remained at the site of injection. DPH had
obviously precipitated at the site of the injection
(21).

Current dosage forms of DPH for oral absorption
result in fairly complete bioavailability and patient
to patient variability can be attributed to differences in metabolism rates within a given population. The very erratic blood levels and occasional
toxicity of DPH in children (24,25) cannot seem to
be completely ascribed to metabolism. After oral
dosing the blood level maximum of DPH can occur 6-12
hours after dosing, suggesting that absorption takes
place along the whole of the gastrointestinal (GI)
tract. The completeness of absorption in a marginally
bioavailable product will obviously be affected by
the resident time of the drug in the GI tract, i.e.,
transit time. The shorter resident time noted in
children may account for the more erratic behavior
of DPH in children relative to adults.

As previously stated, the aim of this investigation was to determine the feasibility of obtaining
transient pro-drug (7,8) forms of DPH which would
confer acceptably higher aqueous solubility within
the physiologically compatible pH range but once
in the body revert to DPH in a relatively short
period of time. The only previous attempts at
pro-drug forms of DPH appeared in the work of Nakamura
et al. (26-29) who showed that 3-carbethoxy-5,5-di-
phenylhydantoin (III) was a less erratic bioavailable

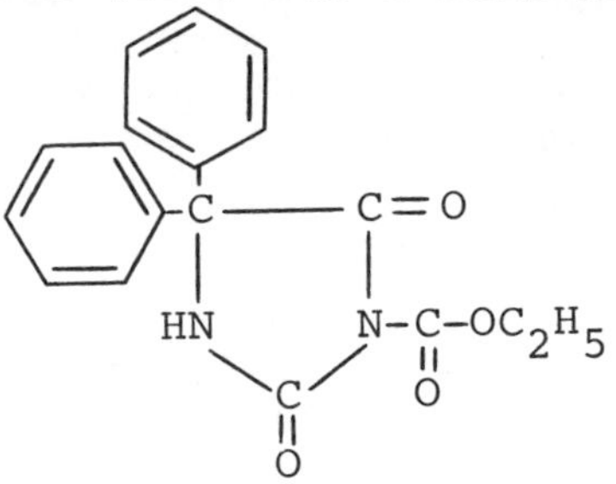

(III)

form of DPH when compared to DPH itself. III, however, was not water soluble so could not be given by I.V. injection.

β-N',N'-Diethylaminoethyl-2-ethyl-5-methyl-2-phenylhydantoate (IV) was recently synthesized and its usefulness as a water soluble pro-drug of mephenytoin (30) was shown.

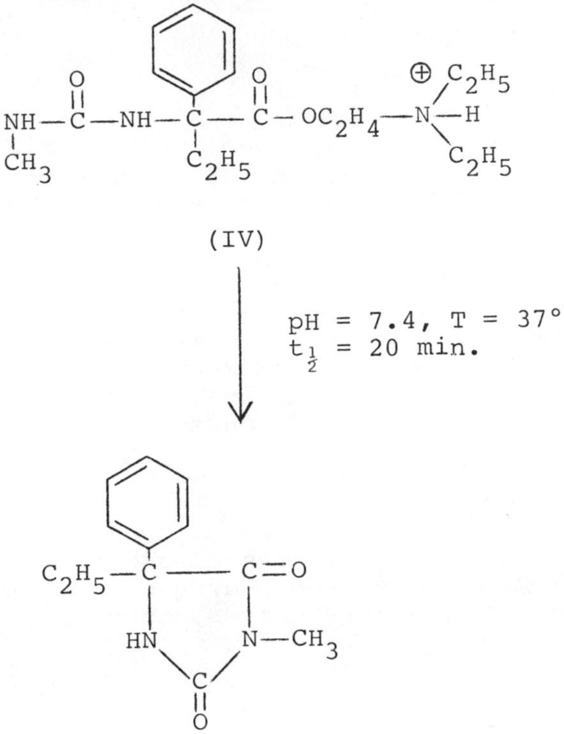

(IV)

pH = 7.4, T = 37°
$t_{\frac{1}{2}}$ = 20 min.

(I)

The synthesis, chemistry, physical properties and formulation problems of a similar derivative to IV but for DPH will be presented at this time.

Rationale

Esters of hydantoic acids were known to cyclize via an intramolecular reaction under basic conditions to their respective hydantoin (scheme I) but no actual kinetic data was available. Kinetic data was available on the cyclization of esters of the related O-ureidobenzoic acid in water in the neutral to alka-line pH range (31). Intramolecular cyclizations had been postulated as a means of latentiation by Levine

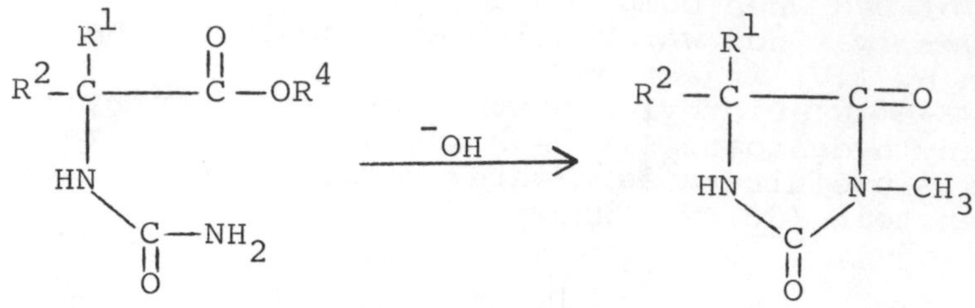

$$R^2 - \underset{\underset{HN}{|}}{\overset{\overset{R^1}{|}}{C}} \underset{}{\longrightarrow} \overset{O}{\overset{||}{C}} - OR^4$$

$$\underset{\overset{|}{C} - NH_2}{\overset{|}{\underset{O}{||}}}$$

$$\xrightarrow{\;^-OH\;}$$

Scheme I

et al. (32) in their work on the conversions of ω-haloalkylamines to their quaternary analogs. In the past,
many derivatives of drugs formed through an ester linkage have been dependent on enzymatic reactions to release the parent compound (33,34). The cyclizations of
the esters of hydantoic acid are intramolecular reactions and these are known to be many orders of magnitude faster than their intermolecular equivalent. This
forms a basis for the formation of the parent drug from
its pro-drug which is not dependent on enzymatic mediation.

Procedure and Results

Because of the apparent success of compound IV in
producing a water soluble pro-drug of I a similar derivative to IV but for DPH was synthesized. The compound of interest was V.

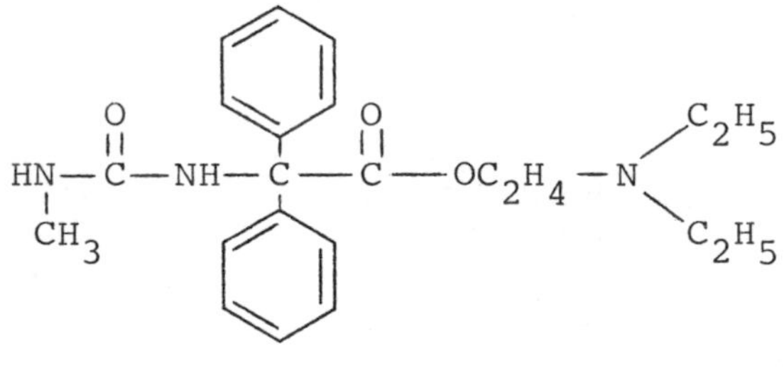

(V)

The synthesis of V was accomplished via the
following procedure and pathway. The first step involved the reaction of 2,2-diphenylglycine with ethyl-
chloroformate under aqueous alkaline conditions. Initially the synthesis of 2,2-diphenylglycine was accomplished by the method of Duschinsky (35) which involved
the actual hydrolysis of DPH in 20% sodium hydroxide

in an autoclave under a nitrogen atmosphere at 180-190° for 24 hours. The synthesis of 2,2-diphenyl-glycine <u>via</u> other procedures such as those found in <u>Organic Synthesis</u>, Coll. vol. 3, pp. 88-91, 1965 met with only partial success. The inexpensive and relatively simple synthesis of DPH meant that it was used as a primary source of 2,2-diphenylglycine. 2,2-Diphenylglycine was subsequently obtained from a commercial source (J. T. Baker and Co.) which apparently also used the hydrolysis of DPH as its method of preparation.

<u>Step I</u>. 2,2-Diphenylglycine (VI), 68.1 g (0.3 moles), was placed in a 2 liter erlenmeyer flask and dissolved in 700 ml 1 N NaOH. While stirring vigorously, 25 ml of ethylchloroformate (VII) and 100 ml of water was added. The reaction mixture was maintained at a temperature of 20-25° by periodically submerging in an ice bath. The pH of the reaction mixture was maintained at 11 or above by periodic additions of NaOH pellets. After 25-30 minutes, another 25 ml of VII and 100 ml of H_2O was again added and the pH continuously adjusted with NaOH pellets. This process was repeated until 250 ml (283.8 g, 2.6 moles) of VII had been added. The reaction mixture was stirred an additional two hours (total reaction time ∿6½ hours) at room temperature. The product, VIII, of the reaction was then isolated as follows:

The reaction mixture was extracted twice with ether (first with a volume of ether equal to the volume of the aqueous reaction mixture and second with one-half the volume of the aqueous reaction mixture). The aqueous layer was transfered to a large beaker and slowly acidified with concentrated HCl (<u>NOTE</u>: The acid must be added slowly to prevent excess foaming and loss of the product.) to a pH of 0 to 1. At this point, considerable solid material separated.

The acidified aqueous mixture was then extracted with ether in the same manner as above. The ether layers were dried over anhydrous sodium sulfate, filtered, and evaporated with the aid of a rotary evaporator to yield a clear, light-yellow colored, and viscous oil. The oil slowly (1-2 hours) crystallized upon standing at room temperature. The crystals were suspended in petroleum ether, filtered, and washed with petroleum ether.

The reaction is outlined on the following page and usually resulted in approximately 75% of the of the theoretical yield. Compound VIII or

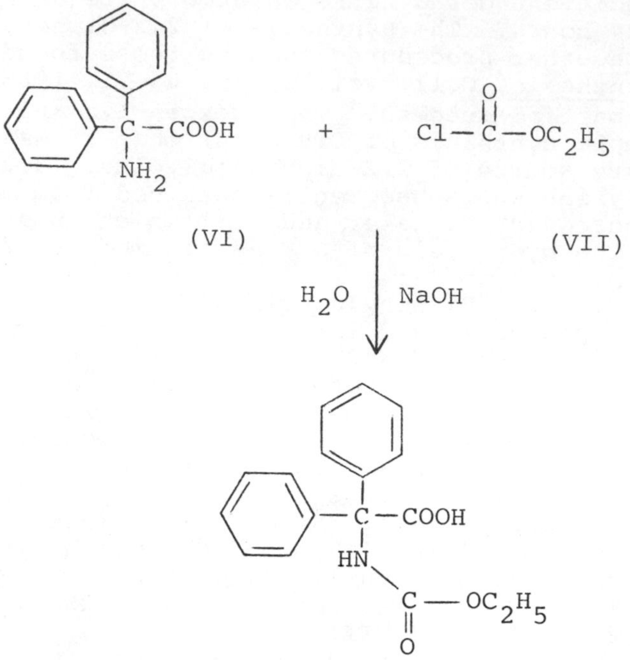

(VI)   +   (VII)

H_2O | NaOH

(VIII)

N-carbethoxy-2,2-diphenylglycine was found to have
a melting point of 150-153°.
    Step II.   VIII, 60 g (0.2 moles) was placed
in a round-bottomed flask fitted with a magnetic
stirrer and reflux condenser and 200 ml (328 g,
7.75 moles) of clear, colorless thionyl chloride was
added. The mixture was slowly warmed to approximately
80° and allowed to reflux for one hour.
    After the reaction mixture was cooled, the ex-
cess thionyl chloride was removed resulting in a
white to light yellow solid (IX). IX was thoroughly
washed with petroleum ether until all traces of
yellow color and thionyl cloride odor were removed.
    The reaction sequence is outlined on the
following page and usually results in 95-100% of the
theoretical yield: The melting point of 4,4-diphenyl-
2,5-oxazolidinedione (IX) was found to be 165-6°.
    Step III.   IX, 50.6 g (0.2 moles), was placed
in a 500 ml 3-necked distilling flask fitted with
a source of HCl gas, an exhaust tube, a magnetic
stirrer, and an oil bath as shown in the sketch on
the following page.

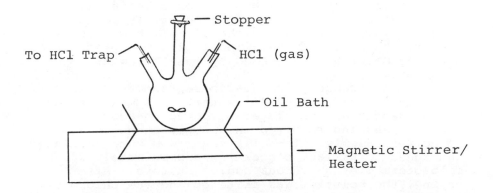

(VIII)   (IX)

After the addition of IX, the flask was
flushed with HCl (gas) and 27.5 ml (24.6 g, 0.21
moles) of N,N-diethylaminoethanol was added. The
stopper was replaced and the HCl (gas) flow restarted
immediately. The mixture was then lowered into an
oil bath at 98-105°, and allowed to react for 15
minutes under a continuous blanket of HCl gas. At
the end of 15 minutes, evolution of carbon dioxide
ceased and a clear oily liquid resulted.

The flask was removed from the oil bath and allowed to cool until the reaction mixture temperature
was below 60°.

The cooled reaction mixture was dissolved in
250 ml chloroform and filtered. A white crystalline
material identified as the dihydrochlroide of β-N',N'-
diethylaminoethyl-2,2-diphenylglycinate (X) was

occasionally observed at this point. This material
may be saved by washing thoroughly with chloroform,
filtering, and adding it to the chloroform solution
of X immediately prior to the NaOH extraction
procedure below.

The chloroform filtrate was placed on a rotary
evaporator and approximately 50 ml of chloroform were
removed. Any excess HCl dissolved in the reaction
mixture was removed by this procedure. The remaining chloroform "reaction mixture" solution was
then extracted with aqueous NaOH until the aqueous
layer had a pH $\geq$ 11. Each fraction (aqueous and organic) was back-extracted and the chloroform layers
combined with anhydrous sodium sulfate.

After drying, the solution was filtered and the
chloroform removed with the aid of a rotary evaporator.
The resulting clear yellow oil should be nearly pure
X as the free base. The oily product may contain
unreacted N,N-diethylaminoethanol, which was readily
detected by NMR. If the aminoalcohol was present
the oily material was washed by the following
procedure:

To the product, in a large separatory funnel,
was added 250 ml cold ($\sim$4°) water. The mixture was
shaken gently and the layers allowed to separate.
Vigorous shaking resulted in a emulsion which separated very slowly. The oily layer was then separated
and added to a flask containing approximately 200 ml
chloroform over anhydrous sodium sulfate. After
drying, the solution was filtered and the chloroform
removed on the rotary evaporator. The resulting oil
was X.

The reaction sequence for step III is outlined
on the following page and usually resulted in 95-100%
of the theoretical yield:

Step IV. X, approximately 65 g, was dissolved
in 170 ml glacial acetic acid. The solution was
stirred in an ice bath until a clear solution resulted. While vigorously stirring the acetic solution, 17.8 g (0.22 moles) potassium isocyanate was
gradually added. The solution was allowed to stir
for 15 minutes in the ice bath and then an additional
three hours at room temperature.

The product β-N',N'-diethylaminoethyl-2,2-
diphenylhydantoate (XI) was isolated as the HSO_4^-
salt by the following procedure:

After three hours stirring at room temperature,
125 ml methanol was added to the reaction mixture.
To a separate 125 ml portion of methanol, 16.7 ml
(30 g, 0.3 moles) concentrated (98%) sulfuric

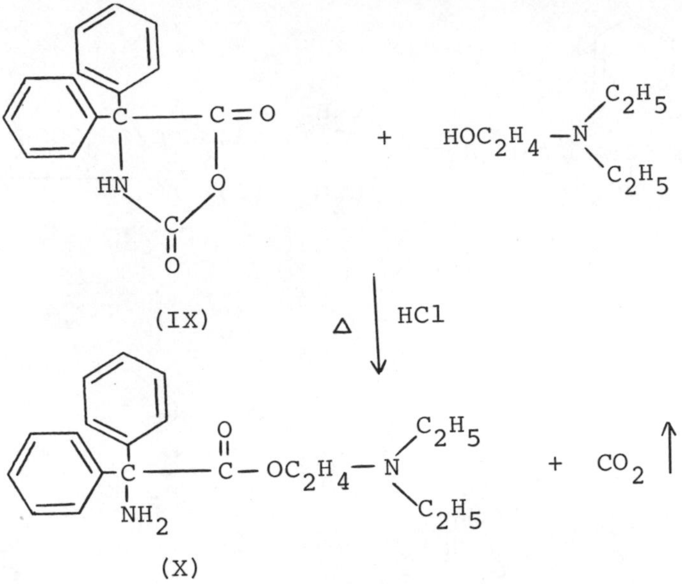

(IX)

Δ | HCl

(X)

acid was carefully added. After the sulfuric
acid/methanol solution had cooled to room temperature, it was added to the methanol reaction mixture
solution with vigorous stirring. The HSO_4^- salt of
product, XI, was then precipitated by the addition
of ether. (Ether was added until no further precipitation occurred. Up to 2 liters of ether may be
required.)

The reaction sequence is outlined on the following page:
The HSO_4^- salt (XI) was converted to the $SO_4^=$ salt
(XII) by the following procedure:
Product XI, 47 g (0.1 mole), was dissolved in
1500 ml water (a clear solution may not result if
product, XI, was impure). Ammonium sulfate, 1425 g,
was dissolved in 2000 ml water and the solution
filtered. The solution of XI was then filtered
into the same flask and the mixture stirred. After
crystallization had commenced, the flask was cooled
to 0-5° and left for 3-4 hours at this temperature
or stored overnight in a refrigerator.

The crystals were recovered by filtration. After
the crystals had been dried on the filter, the
crystals were added to 10 ml of the water. The mixture was stirred thoroughly and the water removed by
vacuum filtration.

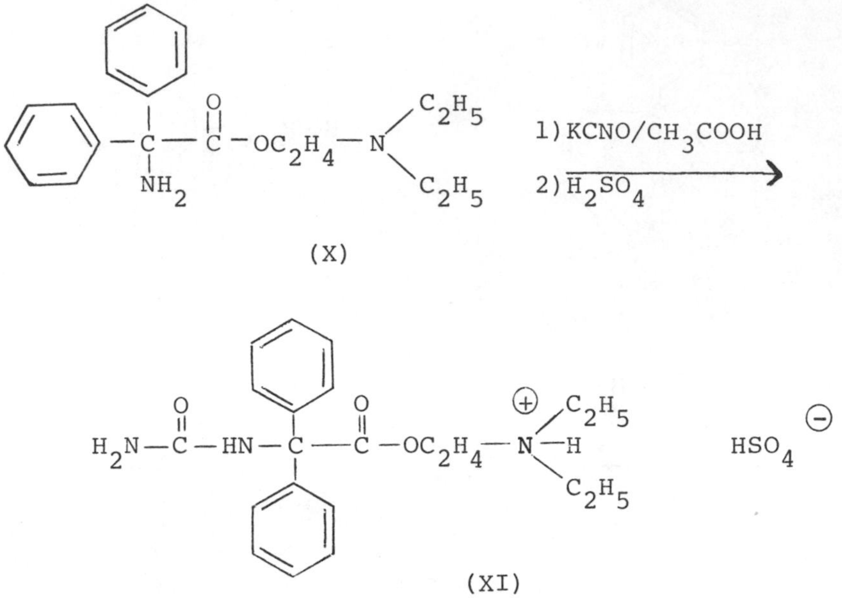

(X)

(XI)

After all apparent traces of moisture had been removed, the crystals were transferred to a flask containing 750 ml of 95% ethanol and stirred thoroughly. At this stage, a clear solution may not result due to the presence of $(NH_4)_2SO_4$. The solution was filtered and the product XII was precipitated by the addition of ether (approximately 2 liters was required). The ethanol/ether solution was stirred for several hours or overnight at room temperature and the crystalline product recovered by filtration.

The percentage yield in the final conversion to product XII was usually quite low (30-50%). It should be pointed out that this step could be improved by a recycling of the aqueous solution.

Compound, XII, or the hemi-sulfate salt of β-N', N'-diethylaminoethyl-2,2-diphenylhydantoate will be referred to as Pro-DPH for convenience; this was the derivative used in all subsequent stability and animal studies.

Table I gives the melting points, molecular weights, % equivalent of DPH and solubility of a number of β-N',N'-diethylaminoethyl-2,2-diphenyl-hydantoate salts at 25° in water. The superior aqueous solubility of the hemi-sulfate salt made it the candidate of choice for initial screening for anticonvulsant activity. Note, that DPH has a solubility of approximately 2 mg/100 ml

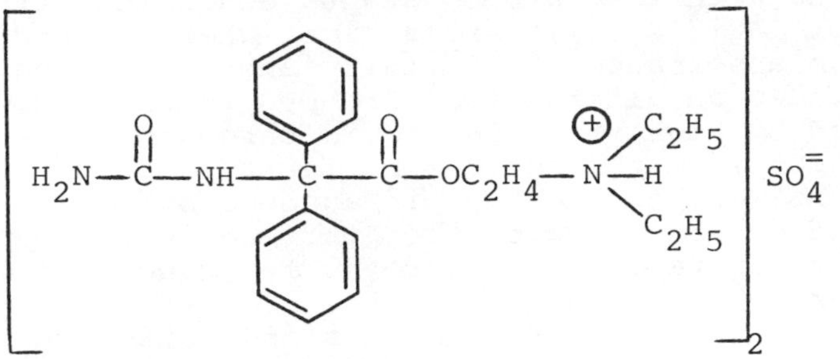

(XII)

or 0.02 mg/ml in aqueous solution at pH << pK_a at 25° which means that the increase in aqueous solubility of Pro-DPH over DPH is about a factor of 15,000 or 9,000 in terms of DPH equivalents.

Table I

Some physical properties of various salt forms of β-N',N'-diethylaminoethyl-2,2-diphenylhydantoate.

Salt	Mol. Wt.	%Equivalence of Diphenyl-hydantoin	Melting Pt.	Solu-bility * at 25° C
HNO_3	432	58.3	173° (dec)	22 mg/ml
HCL	405.5	62.1	188°	23 mg/ml
Salicylate	507	49.7	138°	8 mg/ml
Sulfate	837.01	60.28	145°	301 mg/ml **

* Solubility refers to the solubility of the salt itself and not DPH equivalence.
** This gives an aqueous solution of pH ∿ 3.3.

The conversion of Pro-DPH to DPH was quantitative as checked by spectral comparisons and thin layer chromatography. The rate of cyclization of Pro-DPH to DPH was followed at 25° and 37° to simulate storage conditions and physiological conditions. All kinetic measurements were either carried out directly in the thermostated cell compartment of a recording spectrophotometer, Cary Model 14, or in ampoules placed in a constant temperature water bath. The formation of DPH was followed spectrophotometrically at 245 nm with the rate constants determined from plots of log ($A_\infty - A_t$) <u>versus</u> time, where A_∞ and A_t were the absorbances at infinity and time t respectively. As an alternative, Pro-DPH and/or DPH were followed by high pressure liquid chromatography after extraction from the aqueous buffer solutions. All reactions were carried out in aqueous buffered solutions of constant ionic strength. However, no attempts to extrapolate to zero buffer concentration were made.

The observed rate constants and half-lives for the conversion of Pro-DPH at 25° and 37° in aqueous buffered solutions to DPH are shown in Table II. Figure 1 shows a plot of log k_{obsd}, where k_{obsd} is the observed rate of cyclization of Pro-DPH to DPH, <u>versus</u> pH. Also shown in this figure is the data for the cyclization of the equivalent pro-drug derivative of mephenytoin and β-N',N'-diethylaminoethyl-5-methyl-2,2-ethylphenylhydantoate the equivalent pro-drug derivative of 3-methyl-5,5-ehtylphenylhydantoin. Note that the conversion of Pro-DPH to DPH at 37° is very efficient at pH 7.4, the half-life is 6.8 minutes, but at pH 3 the half-life is about 130 hours. At 25° and pH 3 the half-life for the conversion of Pro-DPH to DPH was found to be approximately 450 hours and at 4°, refrigerator temperature, the half-life was 4000 hours.

It should be noted that in terms of stability the determining factor in a possible reconstituted lyophilized dosage form of Pro-DPH will not be the loss of Pro-DPH <u>per se</u> but more probably the gradual formation of DPH and <u>its</u> subsequent precipitation as the saturation solubility of DPH is reached. The formation of a saturated solution of DPH will be a function of the initial concentration of the Pro-DPH. Since one mole of Pro-DPH released two moles of DPH

$$\left(\frac{d[DPH]}{d_t}\right)_o = 2k\,[\text{Pro-DPH}]_o \cdot \cdot \cdot \cdot \cdot \cdot \cdot \cdot \cdot \text{(eq. 1)}$$

where $\left(\frac{d[DPH]}{d_t}\right)_o$ is the initial rate of formation of DPH from Pro-DPH, $[\text{Pro-DPH}]_o$ is the initial concentration of Pro-DPH and k is the pseudo first order observed rate constant for the conversion of Pro-DPH to DPH under the designated experimental conditions. If $\left(\frac{d[DPH]}{d_t}\right)_o$ is expressed as mg/ml/hr and $[\text{Pro-DPH}]_o$

Table II

The observed rate constants, k_{obsd}*, and half-lives for the conversion of Pro-DPH to DPH at 25° and 37° in aqueous buffered solutions.

pH	37°		25°	
	$t_{1/2}$ (hr)	k_{obsd} (min^{-1})	$t_{1/2}$ (hr)	k_{obsd} (min^{-1})
7.4	0.11 (6.8 min)	1.02×10^{-1}	0.5 (30 min)	2.31×10^{-2}
7	–	–	1.33 (80 min)	8.66×10^{-3}
6	1.8 (108 min)	6.43×10^{-3}	12	9.63×10^{-4}
5	15.5	7.47×10^{-4}	80	1.44×10^{-4}
4	72	1.6×10^{-4}		
3	128	9.0×10^{-5}	450	2.57×10^{-5}
1	100	1.2×10^{-4}		

* not extrapolated to zero buffer concentration.

is expressed in mg/ml then

$$\left(\frac{d[DPH]}{dt}\right)_o = \frac{2k[\text{Molecular Weight DPH}][\text{Pro-DPH}]}{[\text{Molecular Weight Pro-DPH}]}_o$$

. . . . (eq. 2)

$$= k'[\text{Pro-DPH}]_o \cdot \cdot \cdot \cdot \cdot \cdot \cdot \cdot \cdot \cdot \text{(eq. 3)}$$

where $k' = 154 \times 10^{-3} \times 252 \times 2/837 = 9.27 \times 10^{-4}$
hours^{-1} at 25° and at a pH of 3. Table III gives
the calculated zero order initial rates of formation
of DPH from Pro-DPH as a function of initial Pro-DPH
concentration at 25° and pH 3 and the time for
DPH to potentially begin nucleating from solution
(t_{ppte}). The solubility of DPH at 25° and pH 3
is assumed to be 2 mg/100 ml. Table III also assumes
that no DPH was present in the initial sample of
Pro-DPH so the time before precipitation, i.e.,
t_{ppte}, is an optimistic estimate. The value of t_{ppte}
may vary depending on the occurrence of super saturated solutions although this a priori does not seem
likely in light of the strong crystal lattice

Table III

Apparent zero order initial rate of formation of
DPH from Pro-DPH as a function of initial Pro-DPH
concentration at 25° and pH 3 and the potential
t_{ppte} based on Equations 1-3 and a solubility of
DPH at 25° and pH 3 of 2 mg/100 ml.

[Pro-DPH]	[d[DPH]/dt]	t_{ppte} (min)
25 mg/ml	2.31×10^{-2} mg/ml/hour	52 min
50 mg/ml	4.63×10^{-2} mg/ml/hour	26
100 mg/ml	9.26×10^{-2} mg/ml/hour	13
200 mg/ml	1.85×10^{-1} mg/ml/hour	7

of the formed DPH. Figure 2 illustrates the theoretical initial rate of formation of DPH from Pro-DPH.
The time required for DPH precipitation to occur from
solutions of Pro-DPH was determined experimentally
and compared to these predicted figures. The t_{ppte}
did not appear to correlate well with t_{ppte} predicted from the known rates of cyclization of Pro-DPH
to DPH. Table IV gives some of the experimentally
determined turbidity times for various initial concentrations of Pro-DPH.

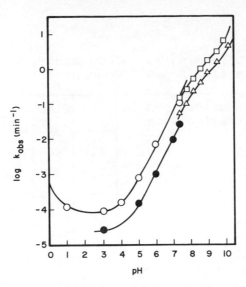

Figure 1. Plots of log k_{obsd} vs. pH for the conversion of Pro-DPH to DPH at 37° (◯) and at 25° (●). Also included are data for conversion of IV to I at 37° (△) and the conversion of β-N', N'-diethylaminoethyl-5-methyl-2,2-ethylphenylhydantoate to 3-methyl-2,2-ethylphenylhydantoate at 37° (□) in aqueous buffered solutions.

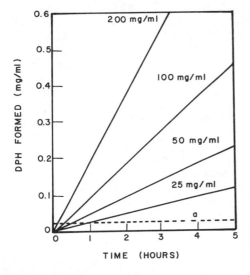

Figure 2. Initial formation of DPH from Pro-DPH as a function of initial Pro-DPH concentration in water at pH 3 and 25°. a = DPH solubility at 25°, pH 3.3 in buffer.

Table IV

Experimental Determination of Turbidity Time as a
Function of Initial Pro-DPH Concentration.

Concentration of Pro-DPH in mg/ml in distilled water	pH	Time for Turbidity Development
83.25	3.6	36 Minutes
83.25	3.7	15 Minutes
124.84	--	1 Hour 10 Minutes
166.5	3.5	2 Hours 10 Minutes
208.1	--	2 Hours 10 Minutes
246.75	3.5	36 Minutes

        To overcome the problem of DPH precipitation, the
following approaches were attempted. The first approach used a solvent in which DPH was more soluble.
This allowed more DPH to form before it began to precipitate out. The solubility of DPH in the current
DPH injection vehicle of 40% propylene glycol, 10%
alcohol and 50% water was 1.07 mg/ml. This meant
that a solution of Pro-DPH of 100 mg/ml and cyclizing
to DPH with a half-life of 450 hours at 25° would
remain clear for 46 hours. This approach would suffer from the problem that some of the toxicity associated with the current DPH injection may in part
be due to the presence of propylene glycol (36,37).
The second approach that could be used (although it
would not be suitable for an I.V. injection dosage
form) would require a sparingly water soluble but
readily dissociatable salt of Pro-DPH. A sparingly
soluble salt (perhaps in the presence of an excess of
the counter anion) could be used to effect a suspension dosage form. On I.M. injection, the absorption
of the common ion into general circulation and subsequent dissociation of the slightly soluble salt should
result in reasonable blood levels of DPH. This technique was attempted using the salicylate salt of XI
(Pro-DPH salicylate) as a model. Pro-DPH salicylate
was found to have an aqueous solubility in water of
8 mg/ml. If 100 mg of Pro-DPH salicylate was suspended in one ml of water the amount of dissolved
Pro-DPH salicylate would be 8 mg, i.e., saturation

solubility. The cyclization of Pro-DPH to DPH at 25° and pH 4.5 (the pH necessary to minimize dissociation of Pro-DPH salicylate) has a half-life of 180 hours or k_{obsd} is 3.85×10^{-3} hours^{-1}. The initial rate of formation of DPH or $(d[DPH]/dt)_o$ from this saturated solution would be 0.015 mg/ml/hour, i.e., it would be 1.3 hours before DPH would begin precipitating out. Table V shows the effect of added salicylate anion on the solubility of Pro-DPH salicylate. In the presence of 0.1 M sodium salicylate, the solubility is lowered to 1 mg/ml so that the initial rate of formation of DPH becomes 0.0010 mg/ml/hour and it would be 10.5 hours before DPH would begin to precipitate. The calculated solubility product of Pro-DPH salicylate from this data was found to be $3.04 \times 10^{-4} M^2$.

Table V

Aqueous Solubility of Pro-DPH Salicylate as a Function of Added Salicylate Anion

Pro-DPH salicylate solubility in mg/ml	Conc. of added Sodium Salicylate	Calculate K_{SP}*
8.7	0	
6.8	0.01	$3.04 \times 10^{-4} M^2$
2.9	0.05	
1.5	0.10	

*Since the pK_a of salicylic is ~ 3.0, K_{SP} or the solubility product will not change significantly as the pH increases, but will decrease by a factor of about two ($\sim 1.5 \times 10^{-4} M^2$) at pH 3.0.

Discussion

The synthesis of Pro-DPH was not short but at the same time did not require any high degree of sophistication. On a commercial basis, the conversion of VI, 2,2-diphenylglycine, to IX might be effected by a one step reaction with phosgene rather than the two step approach taken. Obviously the cost of producing the Pro-DPH would be higher than DPH

itself since DPH is the primary starting material and
the synthesis of the Pro-DPH involves at least a five-
step pathway.

The various salt forms of Pro-DPH and their
variable aqueous solubility (refer to Table I) raises
an interesting and often overlooked point. The
original objective of this proposal was to synthesize
a water soluble bioreversible pro-drug of DPH which
could be administered orally, intramuscularly or
intravenously in a physiologically compatible vehicle.
The pro-drug should not precipitate on injection in
the body and should quantitatively revert to DPH.
The solubility of hydrochloride salts of amines for
oral delivery is suppressed by the common ion effect
of endogenous hydrochloridic acid in the stomach.
Also it is not uncommon for the hydrochloride salt
of large hydrophobic amines to be among the least
water soluble salt. As noted in recent disclosures
and in new drugs approved for clinical use, the use
of salts other than hydrochlorides is a welcome assurance that the importance of the counter anion on
the aqueous solubility of hydrophobic amines salts is
being recognized. The choice of a good counter anion
for an amine drug is often difficult to predict a
priori in that the determining factor in the aqueous
solubility of amine salts is often the strength of the
formed crystal lattice in the solid phase relative to
the solvation energy released on solution. Although
the solvation energy aspects of solubility are often
well understood, solid state geometry and stacking
of the crystal lattice can only be determined by
X-ray total structure determination which is of little
value to the pragmatist looking for a quick answer.
Nevertheless, Table I does show that over an order of
magnitude increase in aqueous solubility could be
effected by the judicious screening of more than one
salt form of a suspected pharmacologically active
agent whose aqueous solubility required optimization.

The partial log k_{obsd} versus pH profile for the
conversion of Pro-DPH to DPH at 25° and 37° shown in
Figure 1 reveals the pH of maximum stability to be
∿2.5. The conversion appears to have an acid catalyzed and a specific base catalyzed component as
well as a spontaneous or water catalyzed component.
The inflection corresponding to a difference in
reactivity of the specific base catalyzed reaction
between the protonated relative to unprotonated
form of the Pro-DPH was not noted because the highest
pH studied was 7.4. As noted in our earlier study,
a partial plateauing should have been noted between

pH 8 and 9.5 (30). The pK_a of the amino group in Pro-DPH is expected to be ~8.5-9.0 at 37° (30).

Kinetically the conversion of Pro-DPH to DPH may be defined by equation 4.

$$k_{obsd} = k_{H^+}[H^+]\alpha + k_0\alpha + k_{-OH}[^-OH]\alpha +$$
$$k'_{-OH}[^-OH](1-\alpha) \cdot \cdot \cdot \cdot \cdot \cdot \cdot \cdot \text{(eq. 4)}$$

where k_{obsd} is the observed rate constant for the conversion of Pro-DPH at a given temperature, k_{H^+} is an acid catalyzed constant, k_0 is a spontaneous or water catalyzed rate constant, k_{-OH} is a specific base catalyzed rate constant representing the attack of the ureido anion at the ester linkage of the protonated form of Pro-DPH and k'_{-OH} is a specific base catalyzed rate constant representing the attack of the ureido anion at the ester linkage of the unprotonated form of Pro-DPH. Although with Pro-DPH no sophisticated physical organic study was carried out (that was not the objective of this study) by inference to our earlier more detailed kinetic study of the conversion of IV to I the log k_{obsd} versus pH profile and Equation 4 were consistent with Scheme II.

At pH's greater than 5 but less than the pK_a of the amino group, the rate determining step appears to be the intramolecular attack of the ureido anion on the neighboring ester linkage. This was considered to be the most likely mechanism because of the lack of buffer catalysis (30). The spontaneous rate constant k_0 probably involves the attack of the neutral ureido group again via an intramolecular reaction on the neighboring ester linkage. These reactions of course involve Pro-DPH converting to DPH with the subsequent expulsion of the N,N-diethylaminoethanol leaving group. The minor nature of the apparent specific acid catalyzed pathway which involves the attack of the ureido group on the protonated ester function is predictable in that protonation of the ester function would not be favorable due to electrostatic repulsion. The diminutive nature of this pathway is consistent with earlier hydrolysis studies on other amino esters such as procaine (37) and atropine (38,39), where little specific acid catalyzed hydrolysis was similarly noted. These reactions did not involve an intramolecular reaction but were normal intermolecular hydrolysis reactions.

Table I noted the 15,000 fold increase in aqueous solubility of Pro-DPH over DPH. In terms of DPH

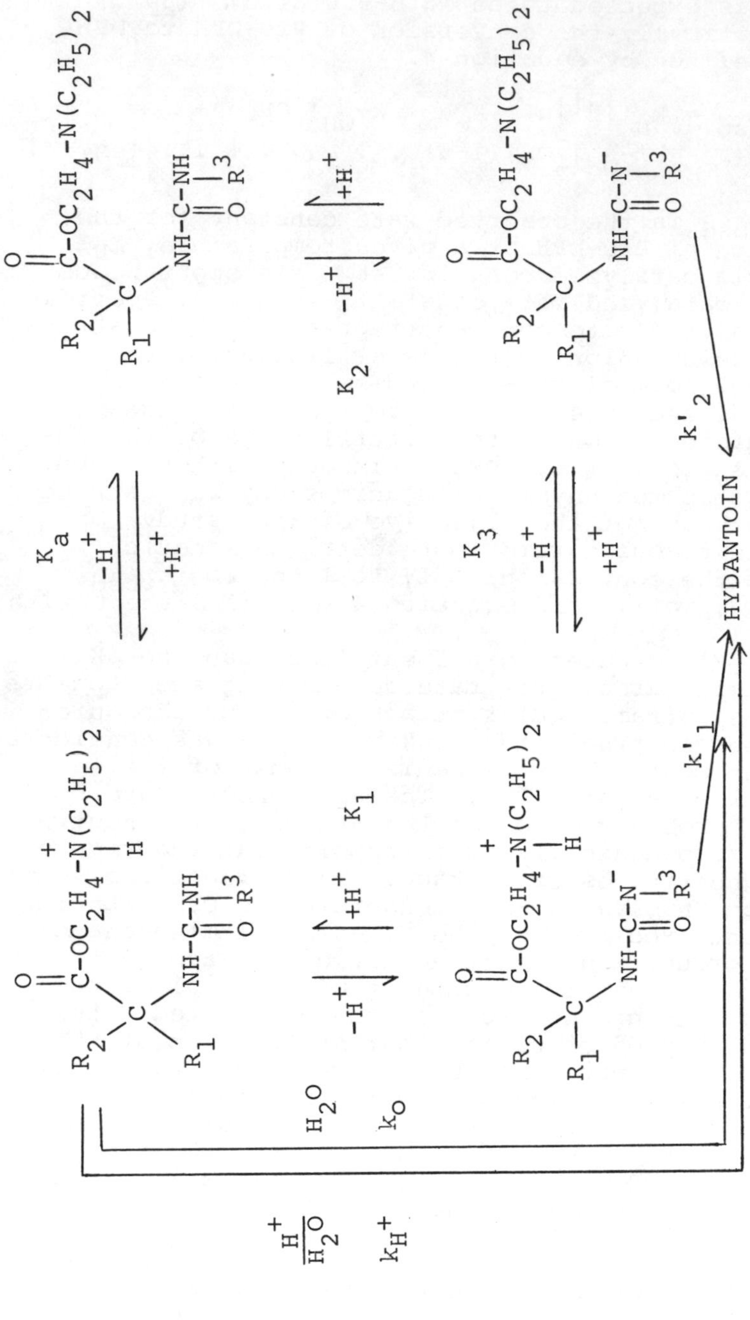

Scheme II

equivalents this was a factor of 9,000. As noted
earlier, the resulting formulation problem, i.e.,
the rapid formation of a saturated solution of DPH
from a sample of Pro-DPH, presented another interesting dimension to the problem. The experimentally determined turbidity times or t_{ppte} as shown in Table IV
as a function of initial Pro-DPH concentration were
not consistent with the theoretical values of Table
III. Increasing initial Pro-DPH concentration should
have led to a shorter turbidity time. This anomalous
behavior could have resulted from two possible
sources: a) The Pro-DPH formed a micellar solution
which helped to partially solubilize the formed DPH
thus lengthening t_{ppte}; b) The Pro-DPH formed micelles
but, in the micellar state, Pro-DPH cyclized more
slowly to DPH than in the non-micellar state. Neither
of these postulated mechanisms were verified but the
fact that Pro-DPH in the presence of plasma was apparently converted slightly more slowly to DPH (see
paper by Glazko et al.) than in the absence of plasma
under the same conditions of pH and temperature suggested that bound Pro-DPH may not be as readily
converted to DPH as unbound Pro-DPH. This finding
would tend to favor the second postulate as the
source of the anomalous turbidity data.

Conclusion

The original objective of this work was to utilize the pro-drug approach to produce a bio-reversible
DPH derivative with good aqueous solubility. It was
hoped that the derivative would have good in vivo
DPH release characteristics (see the paper of Glazko
et al. following) and lead to a superior form of DPH.
A water soluble bioreversible pro-drug of DPH was
synthesized and its physical and chemical properties
studied. The pro-drug was an acyclic form of DPH
which underwent an intramolecular reaction to regenerate the parent compound, DPH. Under simulated
physiological conditions, the half-life for the conversion of the Pro-DPH to DPH was approximately seven
minutes illustrating that enzyme mediation in the regeneration of the parent compound was unnecessary.
The relative stability of Pro-DPH under acidic solutions, pH ∿ 3, allowed a lyophilized powder to be
formed. When reconstituted with water, the extremely
poor aqueous solubility of the gradually formed DPH
did create problems by producing turbid solutions relatively quickly. The effect of the counter anion

on the aqueous solubility of the amine pro-drug was
shown to be an important factor in producing a
satisfactorily water soluble pro-drug.

Other Attempts at Pro-Drug Forms of Hydantoins

In the course of the investigation on the possible usefulness of hydantoic acid esters as pro-drugs
of hydantoins, the acid catalyzed cyclization of hydantoic acids themselves, was investigated in the pH range
0-2. The reaction was found to follow Scheme III. Details of the kinetics and the effects of the R^1, R^2 and
R^3 groups on the closure rate have been reported (40);
of specific interest were 2,2-diphenylhydantoic acid
and 2-ethyl-5-methyl-2-phenylhydantoic acid, the hydantoic acids of DPH and I respectively. The objective of
the study of the acid catalyzed cyclization of the hydantoic acids was to observe if when taken orally, the
closure of the hydantoic acids to their respective hydantoin was sufficiently fast to allow hydantoic acid
to be converted to the hydantoin under physiological pH
conditions. It was found that only in the acid pH region was the closure rate observable. The study showed
that in the pH range 0 to 2 both of the respective hydantoic acids of DPH and I were quantitatively converted to the hydantoin.

The pH of stomach contents in a fasted human is
considered to be in the range of 1 to 3 and the stomach
emptying time for small volumes of liquids is variable.
If the hydantoic acids were to act as pro-drugs of hydantoins, they should cyclize with half-lives at pH 1.5
and 37° of less than 15 minutes. At pH 1.5 and 50°,
the half-life for the conversion of 2,2-diphenylhydan-
toic acid to DPH was 12 hours while the half-life for
the conversion of 2-ethyl-5-methyl-2-phenyl hydantoic
acid to I was 40 minutes. If a three fold decrease in
rate is assumed for a temperature drop of 50° to 37°,
the half-lives for the conversions were well outside
the range where the hydantoic acids might be considered
as suitable pro-drugs of hydantoins.

Reference to 1,3-diacyl-,3-acyl-, and 1-acyl-, derivatives of hydantoins have appeared intermittently in
the literature. As discussed earlier, poor aqueous and
lipid solubility of hydantoins not substituted at the 1
and 3 positions is due in part to strong intermolecular
hydrogen bonding in the crystal lattice. Acylation at
the number 3 position, which displaces the acidic proton, should lead to a reduction in the intermolecular
hydrogen bonding in the crystal lattice. This should
result in the increased lipophilicity of hydantoins as

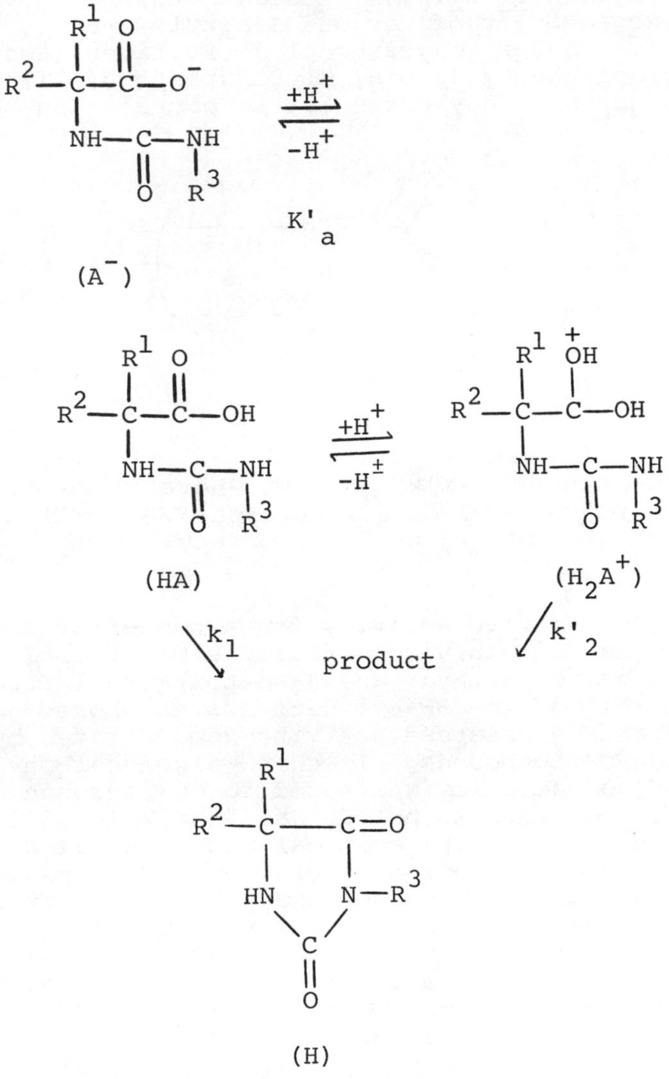

$$
\begin{array}{c}
R^2-\underset{\underset{\underset{\underset{O}{\parallel}}{C}-NH}{\overset{R^1}{\underset{\mid}{C}}}-\overset{O}{\overset{\parallel}{C}}-O^- \\
NH-C-\underset{R^3}{\overset{\mid}{N}H}
\end{array}
\quad
\underset{-H^+}{\overset{+H^+}{\rightleftharpoons}}
$$

$$K'_a$$

$$(A^-)$$

$$
R^2-\underset{\underset{\underset{O}{\parallel}}{C}-NH-C-\underset{R^3}{NH}}{\overset{R^1}{\underset{\mid}{C}}}-\overset{O}{\overset{\parallel}{C}}-OH
\quad
\underset{-H^\pm}{\overset{+H^+}{\rightleftharpoons}}
\quad
R^2-\underset{\underset{O}{\parallel}}{\overset{R^1}{\underset{\mid}{C}}}-\overset{\overset{+}{OH}}{\underset{\mid}{C}}-OH
$$

$$(HA) \qquad\qquad\qquad (H_2A^+)$$

$$\underset{1}{\searrow}^{k} \qquad \text{product} \qquad \underset{2}{\swarrow}^{k'}$$

$$
R^2-\underset{\underset{\underset{O}{\parallel}}{C}}{\overset{R^1}{\underset{\mid}{C}}}-\overset{\mid}{C}=O
$$

$$(H)$$

Scheme III

where R^1, R^2, R^3 = alkyl, aryl, and/or hydrogen substituents.

well as a possible increase in water solubility.

English et al. (41) tested both the in vitro and in vivo activity of various 3-alkyl, 3-acyl, 3-acyloxy-methyl, and 3-alkoxycarbonyl derivatives (see structure below) of the hydantoin, nitrofurantoin (II) against P. vulgaris. They noted little correlation between in

$$O_2N\text{—}\underset{O}{\boxed{}}\text{—}CH=N\text{—}N\text{—}C=O$$

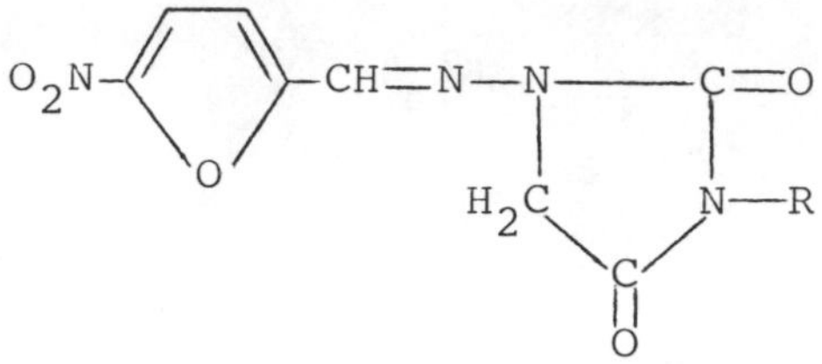

(II)

where R = -alkyl; $-\overset{O}{\overset{\|}{C}}R'$ where R' is an alkyl, aryl or alkoxy group; and $-CH_2OR''$ where R'' is an alkyl or acyl group.

vitro and in vivo activity for a number of compounds. Compounds with in vivo activity similar to II itself were 3-hydroxymethyl- and 3-acetoxymethylnitrofuran-toin. All of the 3-acyl derivatives showed good activity with the greatest activity demonstrated by the C_2 through C_5 compounds. In the 3-alkoxycarbonyl derivatives good activity was noted for C_1 through C_4 derivatives. The authors noted that "the role of 3-substituents in altering the chemical and physical properties influencing absorption, excretion and transport, etc. is recognized". The fact that all derivatives showed the eventual appearance of nitrofurantoin itself suggests that the active medicinal agent was nitrofuran-toin although this was not actually verified in the study.

Reference to 1,3-diacyl, 3-acyl, and 1-acyl derivatives of DPH and 1,3-dialkoxycarbonyl, 3-alkoxycar-bonyl, and 1-alkoxycarbonyl derivatives of DPH have been noted (42-47). A number of these derivatives synthesized by Umemoto (42-43) were subjected to animal trials by Nakamura et al. (26-29) and one derivative, 3-carbethoxy-5,5-diphenylhydantoin (III) has also been successfully subjected to human testing (48-49). Another derivative 3-acetyl-5,5-diphenylhydantoin (XIV) also showed early promise but did not appear to be as effective as III. XIV had a mp of 133-135° while III

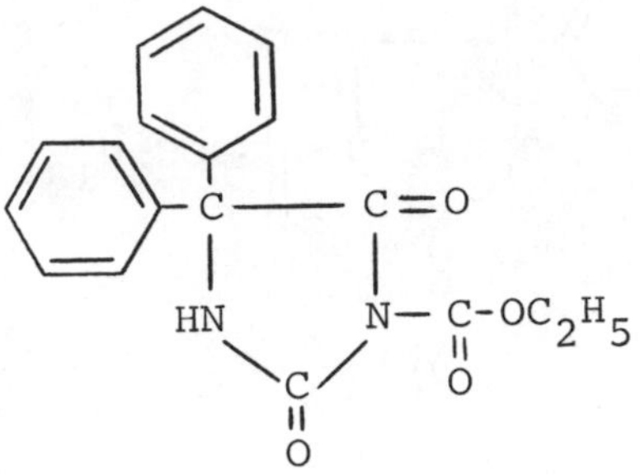

(III)

had a mp of 138-140, i.e., acylation at the 3 position
of DPH caused a decrease in mp of approximately 160°
when compared to DPH. This occurred as the acyl group
displaced the most acidic proton of DPH [pK_a 8.3,
(1,9)] resulting in decreased intermolecular hydrogen
bonding in the crystal lattice. Several studies have
suggested that 1-acyl- and 1,3-diacyl-5,5-diphenylhy-
dantoins had little anticonvulsant activity and were
essentially excreted as 1-acyl-5,5-diphenylhydantoin
whereas 3-acyl derivatives had considerable anticonvulsant activity and in the case of III the activity appeared to be greater than DPH itself. These results
suggest that 3-acyl derivatives are converted to the
parent hydantoin whereas the 1-acyl derivatives are resistant to biotransformation to the parent hydantoin.
Nakamura et al. (26-29) have shown that III demonstrated higher blood levels and higher CNS levels of DPH in
rats and dogs when compared to DPH itself. Both drugs
were given as oral suspensions.

Two human trials comparing III to DPH by Kishi et
al. (48) and Taen et al. (49) were encouraging especially in their conclusions of diminished side effects
of III relative to DPH.

We have recently synthesized a series of 3-alkoxy-
carbonyl-5,5-diphenylhydantoin derivatives with a view
of utilizing the lower melting points and higher lipid
solubilities of the derivatives to effect a soft gelatin capsule dosage form of DPH. 3-Hexoxycarbonyl-5,5-
diphenylhydantoin (XV) has a melting point of 86° and
was found to be soluble and stable in sesame oil, pea-
nut oil, etc. XV was also stable in the bland oils in
the presence of surfactants such as Tween 80. The bio-

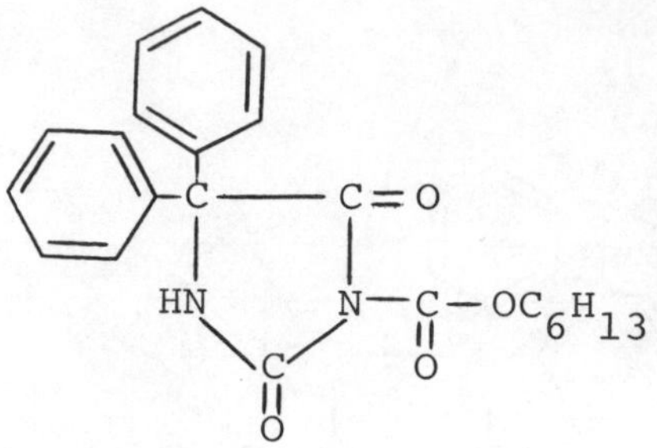

(XV)

availability of DPH from a soft gelatin capsule dosage
form of XV will be reported at a later date.

The hydantoin, 5-ethyl-5-phenylhydantoin (XVI) or
Nirvanol® was marketed as an anticonvulsant drug but
fell into disfavor and was removed from the market because of high toxicity. I is demethylated in man and
dog to XVI and it seems likely that the anitconvulsant
activity of I (see Scheme IV) is, in part, due to its
demethylated product, XVI (50). Therefore, it would
seem that I itself is a pro-drug of XVI.

Pro-drugs of hydantoins are not numerous. This
section has reviewed what derivatives have been attempted with the hope that it might stimulate further investigation into more efficiently absorbed hydantoin
pro-drugs.

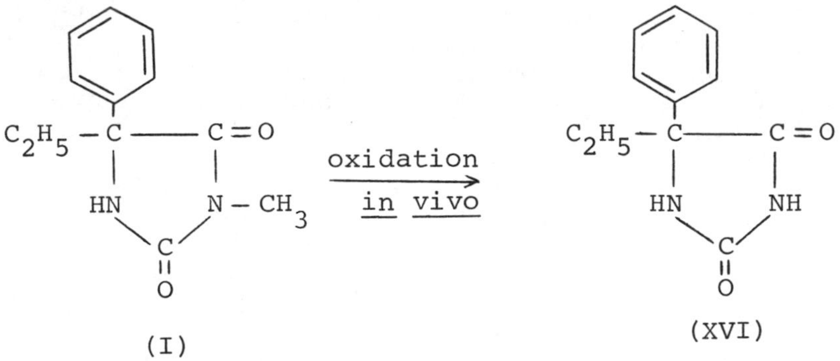

Scheme IV

Literature Cited

1. Arnold, K., Gerber, N., and Levy, G., Can. J. Pharm. Sci. (1970), 5, 89.
2. Martin, C. M., Rubin, M., O'Malley, W., Garaguai, V. F., and McCauley, C. E., Pharmacologist (1968), 10, 167.
3. Rail, L., Med. J. Aust. (1968), ii, 339.
4. Suzuki, T., Saitoh, Y., and Hishihara, K., Chem. Pharm. Bull. (1970), 18, 405
5. Blum, M. R., Riegelman, S., and McGilveray, I., Paper 12 presented to the Basic Pharmaceutics Section, APhA Academy of Pharmaceutical Sciences, San Francisco, 1971.
6. Blum, M. R., Riegelman, S., and Becker, C., Paper 12 presented to the Basic Pharmaceutics Section, APhA Academy of Pharmaceutical Sciences, San Francisco, 1971.
7. Albert, A., Nature (1958), 182, 421.
8. Albert, A., "Selective Toxicity", 2nd. Ed., p. 30, Wiley, New York, N.Y., 1960.
9. Agarwal, S. P., and Blake, M. I., J. Pharm. Sci. (1968), 57, 1434.
10. Glazko, A. J., Pharmacology (1972), 8, 163.
11. Sohár, P., Acta Chim. Acad. Sci. Hung. (1968), 57, 425.
12. "Dilantin®", Formulary Monograph from Parke, Davis and Co., Detroit, Michigan 48232.
13. Atkinson, Jr., A. J., and Davison, R., Ann. Rev. Med. (1974), 25, 99.
14. Frank, J. T., Drug Intel. Clin. Pharm. (1973), 7, 287.
15. Sachtler, G., Drug Intel. Clin. Pharm. (1973). 7, 418.
16. Tobias, D. C., and Kellick, K. A., Drug Intel. Clin. Pharm. (1973), 7, 418.
17. Catania, P. N., Drug Intel. Clin. Pharm. (1973), 7, 418.
18. Chan, N. L., Drug Intel. Clin. Pharm. (1973), 7, 419.
19. Frank, J. T., Drug Intel. Clin. Pharm. (1973), 7, 419.
20. Baldwin, J., and Amerson, A. B., Amer. J. Hosp. Pharm. (1973), 30, 837.
21. Rowland, M., "Clinical Pharmacology", p.27, Macmillan Co., New York, N.Y., 1972.
22. Serrano, E., Roye, D., Hammer, R., and Wilder, B., Neurology (1973), 23, 311.

23. Wilensky, A., and Lowden, A., Neurology (1973),
    23, 318.
24. Lagos, J., J. Amer. Med. Assoc. (1972), 220, 726.
25. Hopkins, I. J., and Rooney, J. C., Med. J. Aust.
    (1969), 2, 278.
26. Nakamura, K., O'Hasi, K., Nakatsuji, K., Hiroka,
    T., Fujimoto, K., and Ose, S., Arch. Int.
    Pharmacodyn. (1965), 156, 261.
27. Nakamura, K., and Masuda, Y., Arch. Int. Pharma-
    codyn. (1966), 164, 255.
28. Nakamura, K., Masuda, Y., and Nakatsuji., Arch.
    Int. Pharmacodyn. (1967), 165, 103.
29. Nakamura, K., Masuda, Y. Nakatsuji, K., and
    Hiroka, T., Nauyn-Schmiedebergs Arch. Pharmak.
    u. Exp. Path. (1966), 254, 406.
30. Stella, V., and Higuchi, T., J. Pharm. Sci.
    (1973), 62, 962.
31. Hegarty, A. F., and Bruice, T. C., J. Amer. Chem.
    Soc. (1970), 92, 6575.
32. Levine, R. R., Weinstock, J., Zirckle, C. S., and
    McLean, R., J. Pharmacol. Exp. Ther. (1961), 131,
    334.
33. Harper, N. J., J. Med. Pharm. Chem. (1959), 1,
    467.
34. Harper, N. J., Progr. Drug Res. (1972), 4, 221.
35. Duschinsky, R., U. S. Patent 2,593,860 (1952),
    to Hoffman-LaRoche, Inc., Nutley, N.J.
36. Louis, S., Kutt, H., and McDowell, F., Amer.
    Heart J. (1967), 74, 523.
37. Higuchi, T., Havinga, A., and Busse, L. W., J.
    Amer. Pharm. Assoc. Sci. Ed. (1950), 39, 405.
38. Kondritzer, A. A., and Zvirblis, P., J. Amer.
    Pharm. Assoc. Sci. Ed. (1957), 46, 531.
39. Zvirblis, P., Socholitsky, I., and Kondritzer,
    A. A., J. Amer. Pharm. Assoc. Sci. Ed. (1956),
    45, 450.
40. Stella, V., and Higuchi, T., J. Org. Chem. (1973),
    38, 1527.
41. English, A. R., McBride, T. J., Conover, L. H.,
    and Gordon, P. N., Antimicrobial Agents Chemo-
    therapy (1966), 434.
42. Umemoto, S., J. Pharm. Soc. Jap. (1965), 84, 504.
43. Umemoto, S., J. Pharm. Soc. Jap. (1965), 84, 509.
44. Takamatsu, H., Umemoto, S., Fujimoto, K., and
    Nakamura, K., U.S. patent 3,161,652, Dec. 15,
    1964; Jap. App., Sept. 12, 1962 through C.A.
    62, 7768d (1965).
45. Garcia Marquina, J. M., and Angles Besa, J. M.,
    Farm. Neuva. (1951), 16, 255.

46. Angles Besa, J. M., Rev. Real Acad. Ciene Exact. Fis. y Nat. Madrid (1949), 43, 193.
47. Garcia Marquina, J. M., and Angles Besa, J. M., Farm Neuva. (1950), 15, 169.
48. Kishi, Y., Fukui, S., Maumara, S., and Aoki, K., Brain and Nerve (1964), 16, 982.
49. Taen, S., Goto, Y., Sekiba, K., and Arai, S., Brain and Nerve (1964), 16, 977.
50. Butler, T. C., J. Pharmacol., (1952), 104, 299.

4

The Metabolic Disposition of a Novel
5,5-Diphenylhydantoin Pro-drug

A. J. GLAZKO, W. A. DILL, R. H. WHEELOCK, R. M. YOUNG,
A. NEMANICH, and L. CROSKEY

Research Laboratories, Parke, Davis, and Co., Ann Arbor, Mich. 48106

V. STELLA and T. HIGUCHI

University of Kansas, Lawrence, Kans. 66044

[5,5-Diphenylhydantoin (DPH; phenytoin; Dilantin®[*])
has been used extensively as an anticonvulsant drug by
oral and parenteral routes of administration. Due to
its low water solubility (about 20 µg/ml at 25° C),
parenteral formulations are dissolved in 40% propylene
glycol and 10% alcohol in water for injection, adjusted
to pH 12 to convert the acid to the sodium salt.] Although this solution has been adequate for intravenous
use, there are clinical indications that intramuscular
use may result in slow absorption and low plasma levels
of DPH. One approach to this problem is based upon the
observation of Kozelka and Hine (1) that[diphenylhydan-
toic acid undergoes ring closure to form DPH when heated with strong acids. However, ring closure of diphenylhydantoic acid proceeds very slowly under physiological conditions.]

Stella and Higuchi (2) studied a number of water-
soluble hydantoate esters and found that cyclization
occurred rapidly in neutral and alkaline solutions at
room temperature, apparently due to a specific base-
catalyzed intramolecular closure. As an outgrowth of
this work, Stella and Higuchi prepared the diethylami-
noethanol ester of diphenylhydantoic acid, first as the
nitrate salt, and later as the hemisulfate (Pro-DPH).
These preparations were tested in the Parke-Davis Laboratories, and preliminary observations on metabolic
disposition were reported elsewhere (3). The structure
of this compound is shown in Figure 1.

Some Properties of Pro-DPH

The first preparation available for study was the
nitrate salt, which has a water solubility of 22 mg/ml
(representing the equivalent of 12.8 mg DPH per ml).
However, most of the experiments were carried out with

184

the hemisulfate salt (Figure 1), with a water solubility of about 308 mg/ml (representing the equivalent of
185 mg DPH per ml). This is approximately 10,000-fold
greater than the water solubility of DPH. Both salts
showed good stability in acidic solutions, but were
converted rapidly to DPH via ring closure in alkaline
solutions. Half-life estimates for aqueous solutions
of the nitrate salt ranged from more than 3 days at pH
5, about 11 hours at pH 6, and 30 minutes at pH 7.4.

Analytical Procedures

In order to study the conversion of Pro-DPH to DPH
in biological systems, and to assay for each compound
in the presence of the other, extraction procedures
were devised to separate the two compounds. This was
followed by application of the permanganate oxidation
technic for diphenylmethane derivatives to form benzophenone, and ultimate fluorometric assay of the benzophenone as described by Dill and Glazko (4). The separation procedure is outlined in Figure 2.

Blood specimens were collected with one-tenth volume of 1 M citrate buffer added to yield a final pH of
4.5-5.0, effectively blocking further ring closure of
the remaining Pro-DPH. The blood specimens were
chilled immediately, centrifuged to separate the plasma, and assayed the same day. In a typical assay, 1 ml
of plasma is diluted with 1 ml of water, 0.5 g of
$NaHCO_3$ is added and the mixture is extracted without
delay by shaking for 10 minutes in a glass-stoppered
test tube with 7 ml 1,2-dichloroethane (EDC). Five ml
of the EDC is transferred to a second tube and shaken
for 5 minutes with 3 ml 0.1N CHl to separate the Pro-
DPH from the EDC. The HCl extract (A) is retained for
fluorometric assay of Pro-DPH. A portion of the remaining EDC layer (4 ml) is transferred to another tube
and shaken for 5 minutes with 3 ml 1N NaOH to extract
any DPH. The NaOH extract (B) is also retained for
fluorometric assay of DPH. Aliquots of extracts A and
B (2 ml) are then made strongly alkaline by the addition of 1.5 ml of 50% NaOH, 4 ml of n-heptane and 300
mg pulverized $KMnO_4$ are added, and the mixtures are
heated on a steam bath for 30 minutes in glass-stoppered tubes. The benzophenone produced in this step is
extracted into the n-heptane layer, a 3 ml portion is
shaken with 1 ml conc. sulfuric acid, and the fluores-
cence is read in a spectrophotofluorometer at 360/490
nm as described in our earlier report (4).

Tissue specimens were frozen on blocks of dry ice
immediately upon removal, weighed, and 10% (wt/vol)

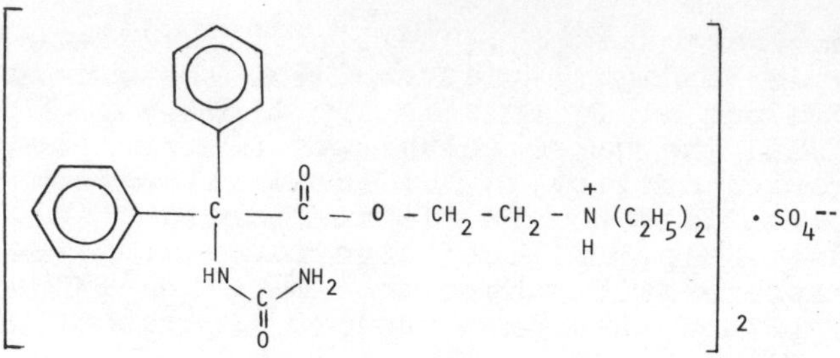

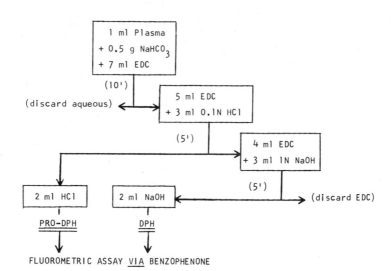

MOLECULAR WEIGHT (SULFATE SALT) = 837.01

SOLUBILITY (WATER) = 308 MG/ML (pH = 3.3)

DPH EQUIVALENTS = 60.28% OF SULFATE SALT.

Figure 1. Chemical structure of Pro-DPH sulfate (N-carbamoyl-2,2-diphenylglycine,2-(diethylamino)ethyl ester, hemisulfate)

Journal of Clinical Chemistry

Figure 2. Extraction scheme for separation of Pro-DPH and DPH. The extracts are then subjected to permanganate oxidation to form benzophenone, which is assayed by the fluorometric technicque. described elsewhere (4).

homogenates were prepared with pH 4.5 citrate buffer
(0.2M). All assay results were expressed in terms of
DPH equivalents. Fluorometer readings were directly
proportional to concentrations of DPH and Pro-DPH over
a wide range. However, with known standards of DPH and
Pro-DPH, about 5% of the DPH was picked up in the Pro-
DPH assay, and about 5% of the Pro-DPH was picked up in
the DPH assay. Nevertheless, this technic provided information which was not available in any other way.

Conversion of Pro-DPH to DPH in Buffers and in Plasma

As an example of the application of this assay
procedure to stability studies in vitro, Pro-DPH sulfate in a final concentration equivalent to 4 µg DPH
per ml was added to 10 ml pH 7.8 phosphate buffer
(0.2M) at 25°C and 37°C. Volumes of 0.5 ml were removed by pipette at frequent intrevals, and transferred
to 2.5 ml volumes of 0.2M citrate buffer at pH 4 to
stop ring closure. The results of the assays for Pro-
DPH and DPH are shown in Figure 3. The apparent half-
life of Pro-DPH at 25°C was about 1 hour, whereas at
37°C the half-life was only 8 minutes. A similar trial
was run with rat plasma plus pH 7.8 phosphate buffer,
with the results shown in Figure 4. Here the apparent
half-life of the Pro-DPH was about 50 minutes at 25°C,
and 10 minutes at 37°C. DPH levels showed a corresponding increase, indicating essentially complete conversion of the Pro-DPH to DPH.

Plasma Levels in Rats

Albino rats receiving intramuscular doses of Pro-
DPH nitrate equivalent to 45 mg DPH per Kg body weight
produced the plasma levels shown in Figure 5. The initial plasma levels fell off quite rapidly, with a half-
life of about 20 minutes, extending out to 1 hour in
later time periods. The initial drop in plasma levels
appears to be due to redistribution of the Pro-DPH into
the tissues, as well as to conversion to DPH by ring
closure. Assay of the muscle injection sites at different time period after dosing indicated rapid absorption of Pro-DPH, with removal of 50% of the drug in
about 15 minutes. The plasma DPH levels rose rapidly
to a fairly flat plateau (6-8 µg/ml) over the 1 to 4
hour period after dosing. Parallel experiments with 45
mg/Kg intramuscular doses of commercially available DPH
in rats produced the plasma levels shown as a broken
line in Figure 5. Although the plasma levels of DPH
after dosing with DPH were somewhat higher than those

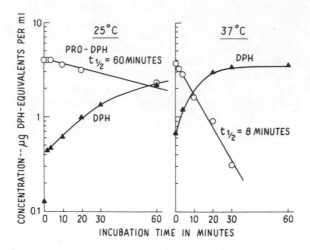

Figure 3. *Conversion of Pro-DPH sulfate to DPH in pH 7.8 phosphate buffer at 25 and 37°C*

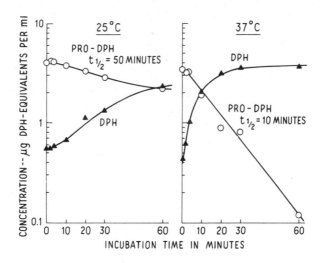

Figure 4. *Conversion of Pro-DPH sulfate to DPH in rat plasma buffered to pH 7.8 at 25 and 37°C*

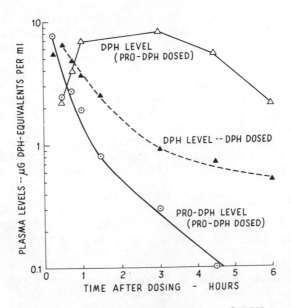

Figure 5. Plasma levels of Pro-DPH and DPH in rats following intramuscular doses of Pro-DPH nitrate (solid lines) and DPH (broken line). DPH assays (△), Pro-DPH assays (○). Doses as DPH-equivalents per kg body weight were 45 mg/kg.

resulting from the administration of Pro-DPH, 15 to 30
minutes after dosing, they fell below the DPH levels
obtained with Pro-DPH in later time periods.

Rat plasma levels resulting from peroral administration of Pro-DPH sulfate in doses equivalent to 50 mg
DPH per Kg body weight are shown in Figure 6. The Pro-
DPH levels reached a peak at or before the 15 minute
sampling time, and then fell rapidly due to tissue distribution and conversion to DPH. The plasma DPH levels
reached a peak of 8-9 µg/ml 2 hours after dosing, at a
time when plasma Pro-DPH levels were quite low. This
could occur only with return of DPH to the plasma from
the tissue depots where Pro-DPH had accumulated, thus
providing a mechanism for extending the duration of DPH
plasma levels in the rat. With orally administered DPH
at the same dose level, absorption from the gastro-intestinal tract was relatively slow, with considerably
lower plasma levels (1-2 µg/ml) appearing 8 to 12 hours
after dosing. Since the plasma half-life of DPH in
rats (< 2 hours) is much shorter than in man (> 15
hours), this factor is not expected to provide a therapeutic advantage over DPH in human subjects.

Plasma Levels in Dogs

Plasma levels of DPH and Pro-DPH were determined
in a series of dogs receiving intravenous doses of Pro-
DPH sulfate equivalent to 7, 14 and 27 mg DPH per Kg
body weight. The results are shown in Figure 7. The
initial plasma levels of Pro-DPH were considerably
higher than those observed in the rats, due to the difference in routes of administration. There was an expected rapid fall in Pro-DPH plasma levels accompanied
by a sharp rise in plasma DPH to plateau levels within
1 hour. These were roughly proportional to dosage, and
they were maintained quite well at the two higher dose
levels over the 160 minute blood sampling period. However, at the lower dose level, there was a noticable
decrease in the DPH plasma levels over the same time
period. These doses of Pro-DPH were well tolerated by
the dogs, whereas similar doses of DPH produced acute
side-effects, such as tremors and vomiting. This is
probably due to the poor diffusion of Pro-DPH into the
central nervous system, as indicated by the tissue distribution studies.

Tissue Distribution Studies

Albino rats were given intramuscular doses of Pro-
DPH sulfate equivalent to 50 mg DPH per Kg body weight,

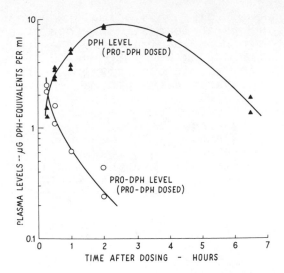

Figure 6. Plasma levels in rats (two per time period) following peroral doses of Pro-DPH sulfate equivalent to 50 mg DPH per kg body weight. DPH assays (△), Pro-DPH assays (○).

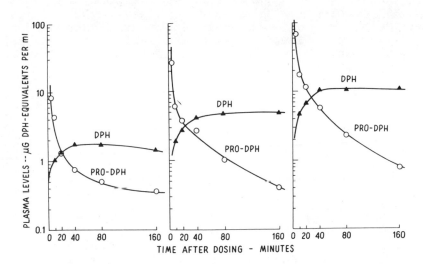

Figure 7. Plasma levels of Pro-DPH and DPH in dogs following intravenous doses of Pro-DPH sulfate equivalent to 7 (left), 14 (center), and 27 (right) mg DPH equivalents per kg body weight. DPH assays (△), Pro-DPH assays (○).

and the tissues in different animals were assayed for
Pro-DPH and DPH at various time periods after dosing.
The results are shown in Figure 8. The Pro-DPH levels
10 minutes after dosing were highest in the kidneys,
lungs and spleen, with progressively lower levels occurring in the liver, heart, plasma, skeletal muscle
and body fat. The tissue levels of Pro-DPH fell of at
a fairly constant rate with an estimated half-life of
30 minutes. Only traces of drug were found in the
brain, indicating that Pro-DPH does not readily cross
the blood-brain barrier. DPH levels in the tissues
showed a steady increase over the 90 minute period of
the experiment, and its distribution was similar to
that observed following oral or parenteral doses of
DPH.

A similar tissue distribution study was carried
out in a series of 5 dogs given intravenous doses of
Pro-DPH sulfate (equivalent to 14 mg per Kg body
weight), and sacrificed at different time periods after
dosing. The results are shown in Figure 9. The tissue
distribution of Pro-DPH was very similar to that observed in the rat, although initially at much higher
levels due to the route of administration. Most tissues had their highest levels 5 minutes after dosing,
indicating very rapid diffusion of drug into the tissues. The Pro-DPH levels fell rapidly for the first
half-hour, and then more slowly with an estimated half-
life of 35 minutes. Again, only traces of Pro-DPH were
found in brain (< 1 µg/g), indicating poor transport
across the blood-brain barrier. However, DPH levels in
the brain rose to 5-6 µg/g in about 30 minutes, in parallel with the plasma levels, indicating entry of DPH
into the central nervous system after it had been
formed elsewhere in the body.

Urinary Excretion

The urinary excretion of DPH and Pro-DPH sulfate
was measured in rats following I.M. doses of the two
drugs, equivalent to 50 mg DPH per Kg body weight.
Urine was collected for 22 hours over dry ice to keep
the specimens frozen. Upon thawing, pH 4.5 citrate
buffer was added to minimize ring closure. Assay results are shown in Table 1.

When DPH was administered, the excretion of unchanged DPH represented 0.05-0.15% of the dose. However, when Pro-DPH was administered, 2.0-3.0% of the
dose was recovered as free DPH. Since very limited
quantities of DPH appear in the urine following administration of DPH, it is difficult to see why such in-

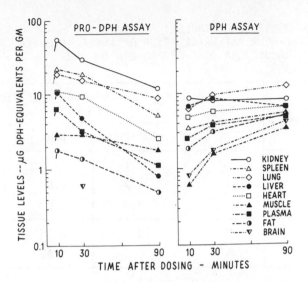

Figure 8.   Tissue levels of Pro-DPH and DPH in rats following intramuscular doses of Pro-DPH sulfate equivalent to 50 mg DPH per kg body weight

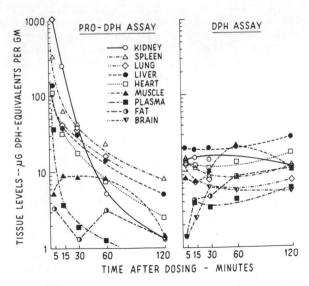

Figure 9.   Tissue levels of Pro-DPH and DPH in dogs following intravenous doses of Pro-DPH sulfate equivalent to 14 mg DPH per kg body weight

TABLE 1
ASSAY OF 22-HOUR RAT URINE AFTER A SINGLE 50 MG/KG
INTRAMUSCULAR DOSE OF PRO-DPH OR DPH

DRUG ADMINISTERED	RAT NO.	URINARY EXCRETION PER CENT OF DOSE		
		PRO-DPH	DPH	TOTAL
		(%)	(%)	(%)
PRO-DPH	1	4.2	2.0	6.2
	2	3.0	3.0	6.0
DPH	3	0	0.15	0.15
	4	0	0.05	0.05

creased amounts are excreted following administration
of Pro-DPH, unless the Pro-DPH itself undergoes ring
closure in urine filtrates. The assays indicate that
some Pro-DPH is excreted unchanged in rat urine. This
aspect of Pro-DPH metabolism requires further investigation, since it is possible that the DPH generated
from Pro-DPH in urine may reach a saturation point,
producing crystalluria or even deposition of crystals
in the renal tissue. The pH of the urine would be expected to be a critical factor in affecting the rate of
ring closure. These and other related aspects of Pro-
DPH metabolism require further examination in animal
studies, especially with repeated doses of Pro-DPH, before this pro-drug can be regarded as a suitable candidate for therapeutic use in man.

Summary

Pro-DPH is of interest because of its high water
solubility and ease of conversion to DPH in biological
systems. Assay procedures were devised to measure the
concentration of DPH and Pro-DPH in the same biological
specimens. Pro-DPH was found to be absorbed rapidly
from intramuscular injection sites in rats and dogs,
and it showed good absorption characteristics from the
gastro-intestinal tract of the rat. The plasma levels
of Pro-DPH fell rapidly due to distribution into the
tissues and conversion to DPH by ring closure. This
was accompanied by the appearance of high and extended
plasma levels of DPH, which were roughly proportional

to dosage. Highest concentrations of Pro-DPH were found in the kidneys, with somewhat lower concentrations in the spleen and lungs; only traces of Pro-DPH were found in the brain. Excretion data in rats indicate that some Pro-DPH is excreted unchanged in the urine, and that a portion may be converted to DPH after clearance through the kidneys. Additional work is needed in this area before Pro-DPH can be cleared for human trial.

Literature Cited

1. Kozelka, F. L., and Hine, C. E., J. Pharmacol. Exper. Therap. (1941), 72, 276.
2. Stella, V., and Higuchi, T., J. Pharmaceut. Sci. (1973), 62, 962.
3. Glazko, A. J., Dill, W. A., Wheelock, R. H., Nemanich, A., Croskey, L., and Higuchi, T., Federat. Proc. (1973), 32, 684.
4. Dill, W. A., and Glazko, A. J., Clin. Chem. (1972), 18, 675.

FOOTNOTE

* Dilantin® is the Parke, Davis & Company tradename for 5,5-diphenylhydantoin.

5

Case Histories of the Development of Pro-drugs for Use in the Formulation of Cytotoxic Agents in Parenteral Solutions

ARNOLD J. REPTA

Department of Pharmaceutical Chemistry, School of Pharmacy,
University of Kansas, Lawrence, Kans. 66044

Introduction

The pro-drug approach can be utilized to improve drug delivery through a number of related but distinctly different mechanisms. These might include use of a pro-drug in attempting 1) to alter the rate of metabolism of the drug, 2) to alter the rate of release from a dosage form or depot site, and/or 3) to deliver the drug to a specific site or organ in the body. The achievement of any one or a combination of two or more of these objectives would be expected to have significant effects on the concentration vs time profile of the drug at the receptor site. Although the technology for achieving any one or more such goals could probably be developed for a given drug substance, a good deal of data would have to be available relative to the metabolism, site of action, toxicity and desired concentration-time profile for that drug in the body. Only on the basis of such information would it be possible to define the specific properties and characteristics that need be incorporated in the pro-drug. Obviously, the application of pro-drug approaches in order to attain such objectives requires that there be both a great deal of interest in the drug and considerable advantage to be gained before one could justify committing the resources necessary for the design and development of a suitable pro-drug.

A more common and presumably more achievable objective, which would involve the use of pro-drugs for improved drug delivery, would be that concerned with the enhancement of the absorption or bioavailability of a drug through some reversible alteration of the properties of the drug. Pro-drugs used for such a purpose would normally exhibit an apparent increase in the solubility or stability of the drug which in turn would

196

allow the drug to be released from the dosage form and
to arrive at the receptor site more rapidly and/or more
completely when employed as the pro-drug form.

The problem of poor bioavailability of certain cytotoxic agents of interest in cancer chemotherapy has
apparently led to a desire by investigators working
with the National Cancer Institute to carry out clinical testing of such agents as intravenous solutions.
This preference for solution dosage forms results from
the current acceptance of intravenous administration of
a drug as representing complete bioavailability (1).
While such equivalence may be argued (1,2), comparison
of clinical activity of different drugs and drug re-
gimes administered in this way would certainly appear
to be superior to administration by any other route or
combination of routes.

Although the use of intravenous solutions in clinical testing of cytotoxic agents seems to be both rational and well accepted, often there are major problems encountered in the formulation of some of these
agents in solutions suitable for intravenous use. Such
problems usually involve the solubility and/or the
chemical stability of the candidate drugs in physiologically acceptable solvent systems. Many of these specific problems may be overcome by formulating as acidic
or alkaline aqueous solutions, by using mixed solvent
systems, by using dry formulations which are reconstituted just prior to use, and by various other completely acceptable techniques. However, on occasion certain
cytotoxic agents present problems for which such solutions are not adequate and these are the types of substances for which the pro-drug approach is most appli-
cable.

The identification and use of a pro-drug system as
the solution to a delivery problem which could be
solved by salt formation, pH adjustment, use of cosolvents, or other simple formulation techniques appears
to be a superfluous exercise and should probably be
discouraged in light of the time and resources which
would normally be required to bring such an approach to
a successful conclusion. Thus when a stability or solubility problem has been encountered, the rational development of the answer to the problem begins with a
series of questions which must be asked and answered
carefully.

The first question to be considered is, "Can the
gross problem be obviated by any of the more or less
trivial manipulations such as pH adjustment, etc?" If
the answer to the first question is negative, the second question is asked. It is, "What are the basic fac-

tors giving rise to the gross problem being confron-
ted?" The answer to this question is usually multifac-
eted and often cannot be answered with complete certainty. Usually the answer requires obtaining and
evaluating various physical and chemical data about the
candidate drug. The particular nature of the data
needed depends on the problem type. For instance, if
the problem is one of the low aqueous solubility of the
substance, then information on the melting behavior,
the solubility in a variety of solvents, the structural
features, etc., are important. If the problem is stability related, then the nature of the degradation
products, the kinetic order of the degradation process,
information relative to reaction mechanism and any and
all other data pertaining to the degradation reaction
are useful. The careful evaluation of these types of
information and similar information on related compounds often allows one to specify with some degree of
certainty the basic factors causing the problem. For
example, the low aqueous solubility of a rather polar
compound which has a high melting point and a low solubility in virtually all solvents could perhaps be attributed to strong intermolecular hydrogen bonding interactions in the crystalline state. This would cause
the thermodynamic activity of the solute phase to be
low which in turn gives rise to the observed low solubility. A second example, involving a stability problem, might be a situation where the data may suggest
that inter- or intramolecular catalysis by some functional group in the drug molecule is responsible for
the rapid degradation.

After answering the second question, one can pro-
ceed to the next question which is, "What specific type
of manipulation of the molecule or system can be accomplished so that the basic cause or causes will be sufficiently ameliorated so as to solve the gross problem?"

Normally the generic answer to this question is
not a difficult one. This is particularly true if the
previous question (relative to the basic causes of the
problem) was answered in unequivocal terms. As an example, a solution to the above described solubility
problem, which stemmed from hydrogen bonding, might be
the disruption of the hydrogen bonding by preparing a
chemical derivative which would be incapable of acting
as a hydrogen donor. Similarly an answer to the stability problem previously described might involve using
some physical or chemical alteration of the system
which would tie up the functional group responsible for
the catalysis of the decomposition reaction.

The fourth and final (and perhaps the most difficult) question to be asked is, "What specific pro-drug
approach can be used to achieve the desired effect on
the properties of the drug substance and yet, while
being sufficiently stable in the dosage form, will rapidly release the parent drug in the body upon administration?" The answer to this question is often a difficult one since it requires that the approach to be
used must satisfy the general aims of the answer to
question three and additionally it must contain a
built-in releasing mechanism which is triggered by some
agent or event encountered upon administration of the
pro-drug. This trigger must dependently and rapidly
allow or cause the pro-drug to revert to the free parent drug.

It appears that there are at least three such potential triggering mechanisms which are encountered in
the administration of intravenous solutions. The first
of these is the various enzymes in the blood and other
tissues (3). If one designs a pro-drug which will
serve as a substrate for one or more of the enzymes
found in the body and if total enzymatic activity is
sufficiently large, then the release of the drug from
the pro-drug will be much enhanced.

Another potential trigger is the event involving
the dilution of the pro-drug formulation upon administration of the solution into the bloodstream. Such dilution results in reduced concentrations of components
and thus causes shifts in equilibria. An example of a
pro-drug system for which this trigger would be suitable is one involving complexation which is subject to
the law of mass action (4).

The buffered and relatively constant value of the
physiological pH (= 7.4) is a third factor which may be
useful in triggering the release of a drug from a pro-
drug. In those cases where the pH and buffer capacity
of the blood is to be used to advantage, it would seem
to be necessary that the 'pro-drug→drug' reaction be
very pH sensitive, and that the pro-drug formulation
used be at a pH value appreciably different than
pH 7.4.

In view of the limited number of triggering mechanisms available one must carefully consider the physi-
co-chemical characteristics of the various potential
pro-drug approaches with a view toward selecting only
those pro-drug systems which will be most responsive to
one or more of the available triggers encountered upon
intravenous administration of the final formulation.

When all of the above four questions have been
satisfactorily answered, the pro-drug system must be

prepared and tested.   Initial in vitro tests will usually screen out many unsuccessful approaches.   However,
the final proof of the utility of the pro-drug approach
selected will necessarily await the results of in vivo
testing.
        The remainder of this discussion is a review of
the concerns involved in the identification and evaluation of some pro-drug approaches used in attempting to
solve problems associated with the intravenous delivery
of three cytotoxic agents.

Case I.   Identification of 9-(5-0-formyl-β-D-arabino-
furanosyl)adenine as a pro-drug of 1-β-D-arabinofurano-
syladenine.

        The compound 1-β-D-arabinofuranosyladenine (I) is
a nucleoside which is most commonly called ara-A.   It
is the 2'epimer of adenosine (II) and considerable interest has been generated in the compound because of
its ability to inhibit the growth of some viruses (5)
and tumors (6).

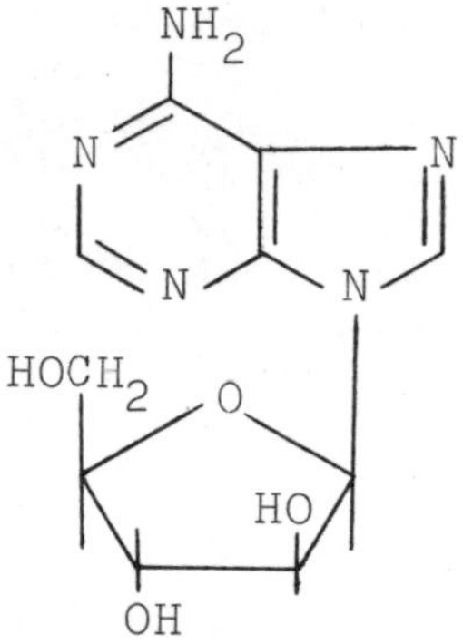

I   II

ara-A   adenosine

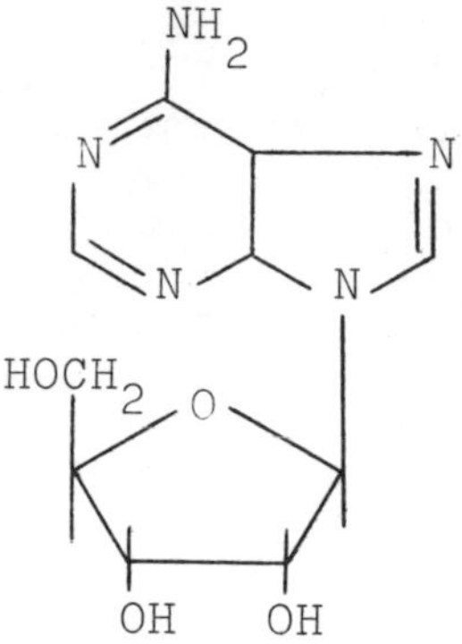

        Some clinical testing of ara-A as a cancer chemo-
therapeutic agent has been attempted but a full scale
evaluation has been severely limited because of problems associated with the administration of the drug.
Human adult doses of 2.5 grams have been suggested and
actually administered as an aqueous intravenous infusion, but the low solubility value of ∿0.5 mg per ml of
water (8) found for ara-A have necessitated the use of
5 to 6 liters of such solutions.   Obviously, such a
large volume of solution requires administration over a
prolonged period of time (9).

Along with the necessarily slow administration, there is a problem of the enzymatic metabolism of ara-A by adenosine deaminase (10,11) to the corresponding hypoxanthine derivative (III, ara-H) which is ineffective in inhibiting tumor growth (12). The biological half-life of the enzymatic deamination reaction is reported to be about 30 minutes (12). Such fascile metabolism, together with the slow administration, makes it impossible to achieve appreciable blood levels of ara-A. Thus a meaningful clinical evaluation of the inherent antitumor activity of ara-A was difficult to make.

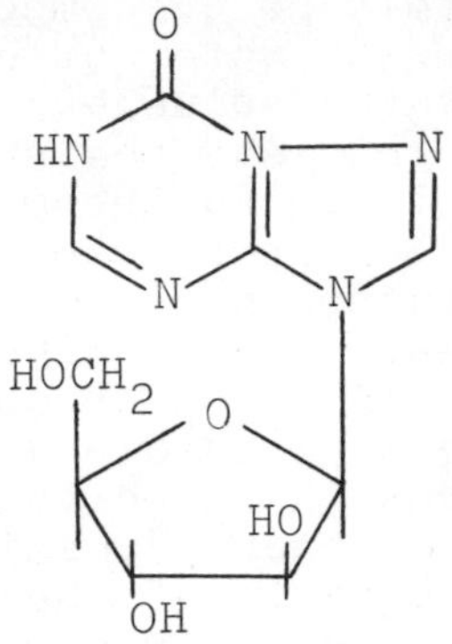

III

ara-H

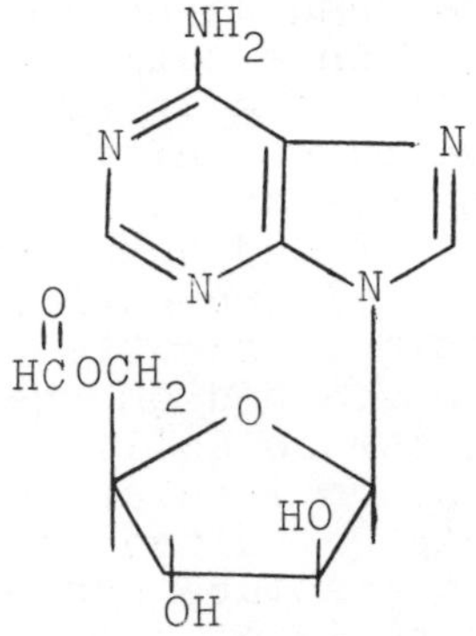

IV

ara-A-5'-formate

It seemed that the most logical and simplest approach to achieving improved drug delivery in this case was to increase the rate at which the drug could be administered. This involved preparing and using a more concentrated solution suitable for intravenous use.

Rather extensive studies aimed at producing an increased apparent solubility of ara-A through the use of mixed solvent systems, agents which would inhibit crystalization, and other approaches had been carried out (13) and proved fruitless. The weakly basic nature of ara-A (pKa ∿ 3.7 (14)) together with its low aqueous solubility and high dose ruled out the use of an acid salt to overcome the solubility problem. Thus, it appeared that an increase in the apparent solubility could not be achieved by simple physical approaches and the possibility of utilizing some suitable pro-drug systems began to be considered.

A comparison of the structural features and some of the properties of ara-A and adenosine, as shown in Table I, brought out some useful points. First of all,

Table I - Some Properties of Adenosine, Ara-A and Ara-A-5'-Formate (14) Water solubility, (25°) M	mp	mol. wt.
adenosine ∿ 0.02	235°	267
ara-a ∿ 0.0018	∿ 260	267
ara-A-5'-formate ∿ 0.12a	∿ 175	295

aDue to hydrolysis of the ester this is an approximate value.

both ara-A and adenosine are highly polar compounds and capable of interacting strongly with water at numerous positions, yet neither is very water soluble. Also, both have rather high melting points, and their solubilities in most solvents is quite low. Furthermore, although ara-A and adenosine are closely related structurally, it is noteworthy that adenosine is more than ten times more soluble than ara-A. The conclusions that were reached on the basis of such information was that the low solubility of these nucleosides was due to strong intermolecular interactions in the crystalline state which resulted in a very low thermodynamic activity for the solute phase. On the basis of the structural features of the compounds, these strong interactions appeared to be due most probably to hydrogen bonding between the various proton donor and acceptor sites in the molecules. The order of magnitude difference in solubility between the two epimers further suggested that the extent of hydrogen bonding changed appreciably with only moderate changes in molecular geometry. Thus it appeared that if it were possible to decrease the intermolecular hydrogen-bonding in the crystalline ara-A, while not significantly decreasing the overall ability of the molecule to interact with water, it should be possible to increase substantially the apparent aqueous solubility. It was anticipated that a decrease in hydrogen bonding could most easily be accomplished by decreasing the hydrogen donor capacity of the arabinose portion of the molecule by substituting non-donor groups for the hydrogen atoms.

At this point in the study it becomes necessary to attempt to define rather specifically a chemical derivative of ara-A which might be used as a soluble prodrug. On the basis of the considerations which follow, the 5'formate ester of ara-A (IV) was initially selected (8).

An ester derivative was chosen since esterification of a hydroxy group would eliminate the hydrogen-

donor capacity at that position. Although an ether derivative would also be effective in eliminating the hydrogen donor activity, the ester was preferentially selected because of its greater ease of hydrolysis, especially in the presence of the various esterases which
abound in blood and other tissues (3). Such enzymatic
assistance could therefore serve as the trigger in the
release of the drug from the pro-drug.

   The choice of the 5' hydroxyl as the site of
esterification was based on the general knowledge that
esters of primary alcohols are normally more easily hydrolyzed than the corresponding esters of secondary alcohols such as are found at the 2' and 3' positions of
ara-A. An additional reason for desiring a derivative
of the 5' hydroxyl was based on the fact that similar
derivatives of compounds related to ara-A were poor
substrates for adenosine deaminase (6,10) and thus the
5' ester of ara-A would probably not undergo appreciable metabolism prior to hydrolysis. While this is an
added bonus it is not an essential factor in so far as
achieving an increased molar solubility is concerned.

   The choice of the formate ester rather than some
other ester was made on the basis of the compact and
relatively polar nature of the formate group which was
not expected to noticeably alter the overall hydrophilic character of the pro-drug relative to the parent
compound. The fact that formate esters are normally
more rapidly hydrolyzed than corresponding homologs was
also important (15).

   The reasons for choosing the monoformate ester in
preference to the diformate or triformate esters
stemmed mainly from a desire to use as simple a system
as possible in order to be able to follow ultimately
the regeneration of the drug. If the triester was to
be used as the pro-drug, (providing it was sufficiently
soluble) random hydrolysis of the esters would potentially result in three different diformate esters which
in turn would hydrolyze to yield three different mono-
esters. This kinetic sequence would then result in the
simultaneous existence of several pro-drug species
which would be present in amounts related to their
rates of formation and degradation. The situation is
somewhat simpler for the diformate derivatives, but
still potentially quite complicated when compared to
that to be expected with the 5' monoformate.

   Ara-A-5'-formate was prepared (8) and the aqueous
solubility was found to change in the anticipated di-

rection. As seen in Table I, the solubility increase
was accompanied by a decrease in the melting point indicating a reduction in the intermolecular interactions
in the pro-drug ester relative to crystalline ara-A.
The approximately 65 fold increase in the molar solubility of the pro-drug in comparison to ara-A meant
that the volume of intravenous solution necessary to
deliver the equivalent of 2.5 grams of ara-A could be
decreased from 5 or 6 liters to less than 100 ml. Obviously such a reduction in volume would allow the drug
to be administered in a much shorter period of time.

Although the problem of the low solubility of ara-
A could obviously be solved by using ara-A-5'-formate,
the potential utility of this substance as a suitable
pro-drug of ara-A depended on its conversion to ara-A
in biological fluids and its stability in an aqueous
solution suitable for intravenous use. In vitro studies carried out in 91% whole human blood at 37° (8)
showed hydrolysis of the ara-A-5'-formate, to yield
ara-A, occurred rapidly. Data from one such run is
shown in Figure 1 where it can be seen that hydrolysis
of ara-A-5'-formate to ara-A was essentially complete
in about 30 minutes. The rather rapid disappearance of
the regenerated ara-A is due presumably to its metabolism by adenosine deaminase (9,10). Nevertheless peak
levels of ara-A corresponding to between 60% and 70%
of the administered dose were achieved. Since both the
rapid hydrolysis of the ester and the deamination of
ara-A are reactions which are enzyme assisted, it is
not surprising that the rates of both processes were
found to be somewhat concentration dependent (8).

The antitumor activity of ara-A-5'-formate, when
tested intraperitoneally in mice innoculated with either Heptoma 134 or Ehrlich ascites tumor cells, was
found to be equivalent to that of ara-A (8) suggesting
that ara-A was regenerated in vivo.

The remaining question which had yet to be answered dealt with the suitability of the proposed pro-
drug in a formulation acceptable for intravenous administration. The aqueous stability of ara-A-5'-formate
was studied and it was found, not surprisingly, that
the most serious degradation problem involved hydrolysis of the formate ester to yield ara-A (8). The effect
of pH on the rate of the hydrolytic reaction was studied at 25° (8) and a portion of that profile obtained
is shown in Fig. 2. At the physiological pH of 7.4, the
observed rate was $\sim 3 \times 10^{-3}$ minute^{-1} which corresponds

to a half-life of about 4 hours.   At pH 4.2 to 4.5,
which was the pH range of greatest stability, the observed half-life was approximately 10 days.

Although it was obvious from the data that the
pro-drug could not be formulated as an aqueous solution with acceptable long term stability, the formate

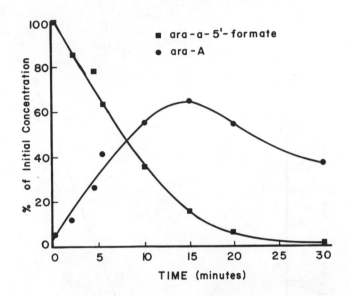

Journal of Pharmaceutical Sciences

*Figure 1.   Plot of the concentrations of ara-A-5'-formate and
ara-A in 91% whole blood at 37° as a function of time, (8).
Initial concentration of ara-A-5'-formate was 2 mg/ml.*

ester was sufficiently (8) stable at pH 4.5 to be used
in a lypohilized formulation to be reconstituted at the
time of use.

Such reconstituted solutions, containing the
equivalent of 30 mg of ara-A/ml (as the pro-drug) would
not be expected to undergo sufficient hydrolysis in a
5 to 6 hour period to produce a saturated solution of

ara-A and thus there would be no problem of precipitation during the time necessary to administer the pro-
drug formulation. Thus it appears in the case of ara-
A that the ara-A-5'-formate meets virtually all the
criteria required of a pro-drug suitable for use in a
intravenous formulation.

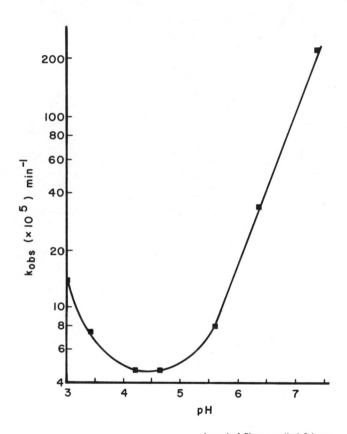

Journal of Pharmaceutical Sciences

*Figure 2. Partial profile of the effects of pH on the observed
first order rate constant for the spontaneous hydrolysis of ara-
A-5'-formate at 25° (8)*

Case II.   Hexamethylmelamine-Gentisic Acid Complexes as a Soluble Pro-Drug form of Hexamethylmelamine.

Hexamethylmelamine (V) is a cytotoxic agent which has commanded clinical interest primarily because of the consistent, albeit low, response rates obtained when it has been used in the treatment of several solid tumors including lung cancers (16,17).

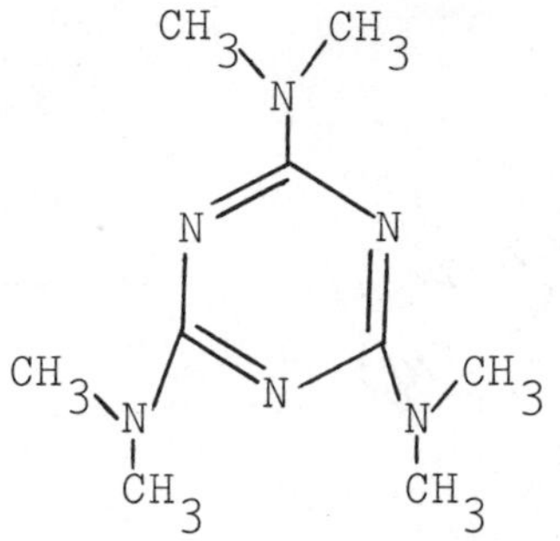

V

Hexamethylmelamine

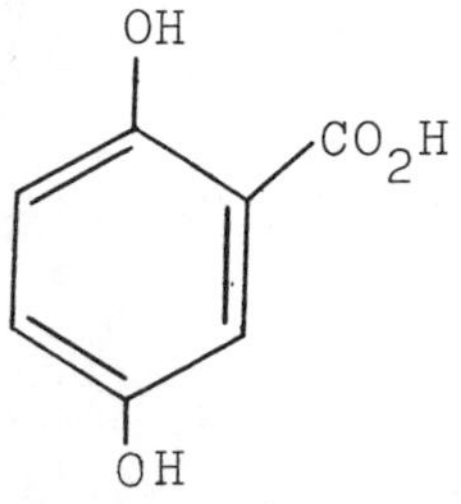

VI

Gentisic Acid

The desire for an intravenous formulation of this drug stemmed from the occurance of the side effects (primarily nausea and vomiting) which its use illicited when given orally (18).   Prior attempts had been made to provide a suitable intravenous preparation based on the use of an acidic solution of the weakly basic drug. However, the combined effects of a pK_b = 9.10, an aqueous solubility of approximately 0.1 mg per ml (at room temperature) (19) and an estimated dose of about 100 to 200 mg (18) resulted in an aqueous formulation of pH 2. The use of this preparation caused serious problems of local irritation and thrombophlebitis (18) which may have been due to either the acidity of the solution or an inherent property of the drug or a combination of both.

In attempting to eliminate or at least reduce the side effects of intravenous administration, a less acidic aqueous solution (pH 3.5 or greater) containing hexamethylmelamine at a concentration of at least 3 mg per ml was requested (18).   Because of its somewhat low solubility in most solvents (see Table II) which might be used as cosolvents together with water, the use of a suitable cosolvent mixture did not appear to offer a good probability of success.   The facts that the compound exhibits good solubility in non-polar solvents

Table II - Approximate Solubility of Hexamethylmelamine
         in Various Solvents at Ambient Temperature
         (19)

Solvent	Approximate solubility (mg/ml)
Water	∿0.1
N,N-Diethylacetamide	30-50
Dimethylsulfoxide	∿5
Ethanol	∿15
Ethylacetate	∿15
Propylene glycol	<2
Polyethylene glycol 400	<2
Chloroform	∿200
Benzene	∿106
Diethyl ether	∿47

such as benzene, chloroform and diethyl ether, while
being considerably less soluble in non-polar solvents
such as propylene glycol, ethanol and especially water,
appeared to suggest that the solubility problem in this
case was not so much due to a low activity of the molecules in the solid solute as it was to a rather high
activity of the dissolved solute in the polar solvents.
Thus one approach to increasing solubility was to decrease the activity of the solute in solution by some
means.

      A method of achieving such a decrease of activity
in an aqueous solution would be through the use of a
more hydrophilic chemical derivative. However, inspection of the chemical structure suggested that the more
apparent chemical derivatives capable of achieving the
solubility increase, such as quaternary salts, probably
would not be useful as pro-drugs since they would not
be expected to readily release the drug under biological conditions.

      The apparent lack of chemical sites suitable for
forming a potentially useful chemically derived pro-
drug resulted in the consideration of complexation as
another method of reducing the activity of the dissolved hexamethylmelamine. A number of characteristics
of the hexamethylmelamine molecule, including its aromatic and its weakly basic nature, suggested that it
would associate or complex with a suitable ligand. In
view of the fact that in the pH 3.5 to 4.0 region, the
apparent increase in solubility which was needed was
only about 5 to 10 fold, it seemed likely that this
magnitude of increase could be achieved through complexation. If the solubility increase desired had been
2 or 3 orders of magnitude or greater, complexation
would not have been seriously considered, since such

large increases are not often achieved by association
of organic molecules in aqueous media.

In choosing a potential ligand for the complexation of hexamethylmelamine two factors had to be considered. One of these was acceptability of the ligand
from the physiological standpoint. The other was the
ability of the agent to interact with the drug. Somewhat fortuitously gentisic acid (VI) was the ligand
initially chosen. This choice was based on the facts
that it is relatively non-toxic (29), has been used
medicinally (21), and thus appeared to be acceptable
from the biological standpoint. Through experience
gained from other studies of the complexation of gentisic acid with heteroaromatic weakly basic compounds
such as caffeine (22), it seemed probable that gentisic
acid or the gentisate ion might be likely to interact
with a compound such as hexamethylmalamine under suitable conditions. Thus the complexation between gentisic acid and hexamethylmelamine was studied and fortu-
nately, as will be discussed below, the system achieved
the desired results (23).

Before proceeding, a brief discussion of complexation and some advantages of such a pro-drug system in
the intravenous administration of drugs is in order.
Complexation normally refers to the association of two
or more molecules of two different compounds in a reversible manner (24). The equilibrium involved in the
formation of a particular complex species may be writ-
en as

$$mS + nL \; \underset{\longleftarrow}{\overset{K}{\longrightarrow}} \; (S_mL_n) \qquad \text{(eq. 1)}.$$

In eq. 1, S and L represent the interacting molecular species, one of which is normally called the substrate and the other the ligand. S_mL_n represents the
complex species formed and m and n are the coefficients
which express the stoichiometry of the complex.

The equilibrium involved may be defined by an association constant K which may be written in terms of
the concentration of the complexed and uncomplexed species as

$$K = [S_mL_n]/[S]^m[L]^n \qquad \text{(eq. 2)}.$$

The properties of the substrate and ligand molecules in
the complex S_mL_n are often quite different from (and
rather independent of) those of the uncomplexed species. In such situations the apparent total molar sol-

ubility, $[S]_T$, may be expressed as

$$[S]_T = [S] + m[S_mL_n] \qquad \text{(eq. 3)}.$$

When the concentration of S is at its saturation value, $[S]_o$, then eq. 3 becomes

$$[S]_T = [S]_o = m[S_mL_n] \qquad \text{(eq. 4)}.$$

It is clear from eq. 4 that if S_mL_n is a very soluble species relative to S then the apparent solubility, $[S]_T$, may be greatly increased by complexation.

Another advantage of such a system, implicit in eqs. 1 and 2, is that in concentrated solutions of S and L, the equilibrium will be poised to the right. Such a situation might be employed in a concentrated intravenous solution dosage form. When the concentrated solution is diluted, as would occur upon the parenteral administration of the solution, the equilibrium would be shifted to the left and rapid and extensive dissociation of the complex would occur. Thus if S was a drug molecule whose solubility was greatly increased by complexation with L, a solution with a high concentration of a soluble ligand L would result in extensive formation of S_mL_n which would result in an increased apparent solubility of S. Such a solution would be physically stable at equilibrium in the dosage form but would release the free drug from the complex upon dilution in blood without any required aid from enzymes or pH changes although the latter may affect the equilibrium in some cases (23).

The effects of gentisic acid on the solubility of hexamethylmalamine was studied at several pH values (23). Phase diagrams of the results at pH 3.5, 4.0, 4.5, and 5 are presented in Fig. 3. In all four cases the apparent solubility of hexamethylmalamine increased as gentisate was added. At pH 3.5 and 4.0, apparently discontinuous curves were obtained and a solid precipitate was formed at added gentisate concentrations of greater than 0.8 $\underline{M}$ (at pH 3.5) and at 1.8 $\underline{M}$ or greater (at pH 4.0).

The reasons for the apparent and unexpected discontinuities were not fully determined but could be due in part to some supersaturation and some very small changes in pH which occur upon precipitation of the complexes (23). In the cases of pH 4.5 and 5.0, no plateau regions corresponding to those obtained at the lower pH's were observed.

It was apparent from the data in Fig. 3 that solutions containing up to 5 mg of hexamethylmelamine per ml could be prepared at pH 3.5 and 4.0. Although it may have been possible to attain an even high apparent

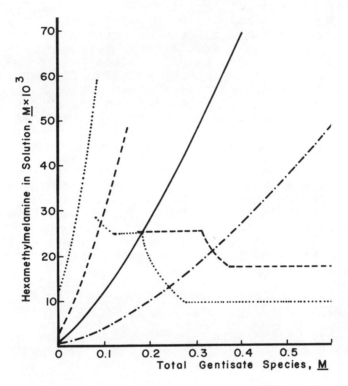

Figure 3. Plot of the apparent aqueous solubility of hexamethylmalamine as a function of total added gentisate species at 25° (23). Key: .... pH 3.5; – – – pH 4.0; ——— pH 4.5; –·–·– pH 5.0. (The data points have been omitted for the sake of clarity.)

solubility for hexamethylmalamine at these pH values, the abrupt discontinuities and the apparent sensitivity of the observed solubility to slight compositional

changes (as indicated in Fig. 3 for solutions containing hexamethylmalamine at concentrations exceeding 2.5
to 3 x 10^{-3} $\underline{M}$) discouraged the use of such systems
which exceeded the plateau concentrations.

At the higher pH values of 4.5 and 5.0, physically
stable solutions containing concentrations of hexamethylmelamine exceeding 12 mg/ml may be prepared. Although a greater total apparent solubility of hexamethylmelamine can be achieved at the higher pH values
shown, the concentration of ligand necessary to achieve
a given value increased sharply as the pH was increased. Thus in choosing the solution formulation it
is necessary to consider the optimum composition with
respect to concentrations of drug and ligand and the
pH. The system which is now undergoing investigation
through the National Cancer Institute is a solution at
pH 3.5 containing 5 mg of hexamethylmelamine and 6 mg
of gentisic acid per ml at pH 5.

A more extensive complexation study than that reported here was made (23) before the preceeding approach was adjudged to be an acceptable solution to the
problem of solubilizing hexamethylmelamine. However,
the present discussion does cover most of the salient
aspects which led to the development and use of the
complexed system as a reversible drug delivery system
suitable for intravenous use.

Case III. Acetylacronycinium Salts and Complexes as a
Soluble Stabilized Pro-Drug Form of Acronycine.

Acronycine (VII) is a cytotoxic substance which
has exhibited activity against a spectrum of tumor test

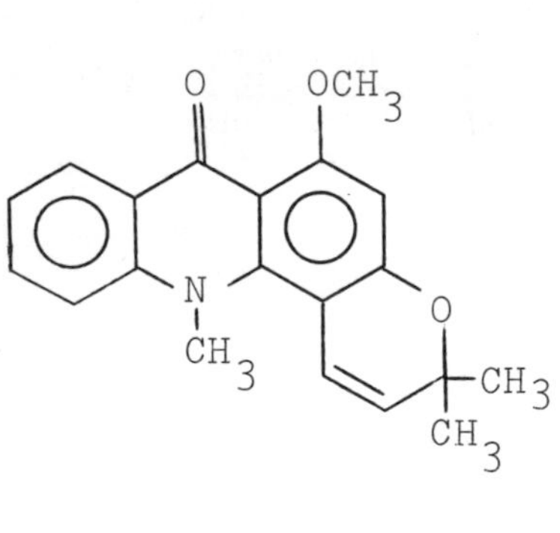

VII   VIII

Acronycine   Acronycinium Ion

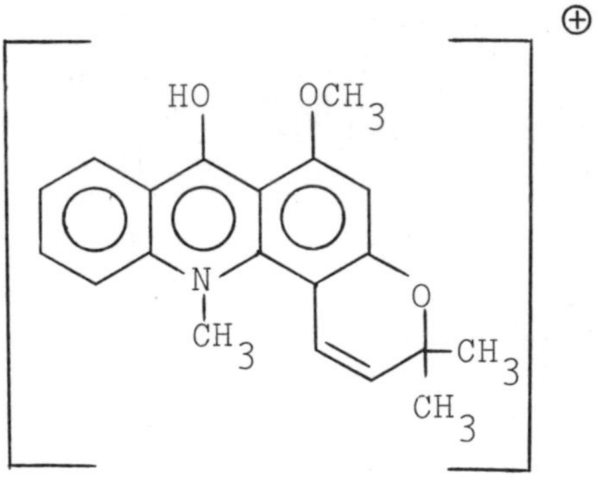

systems (25). However, the low water solubility (∿2
mg/liter)(26) has presented bioavailability problems
and this has made the clinical evaluation of this agent
extremely difficult. The only previously reported attempt (27) made to solubilize acronycine involved the
preparation of a coprecipitate containing polyvinyl
pyrrolidone (5 parts by weight) and acronycine (1 part
by weight). When the coprecipitate was dissolved in
water, an apparent 5 fold increase in the solubility of
acronycine was obtained and the coprecipitate demonstrated enhanced antitumor activity when administered
intraperitoneally as a suspension. Whether or not the
enhanced activity was due to an increase in the equilibrium solubility of acronycine or (as was more probably the case) to an increased dissolution rate of the
coprecipitate relative to acronycine alone was not
clear. Nevertheless, because of the rather large anticipated acronycine dose of 100 to 200 mg, and a desire
for that dose to be contained in a volume of about 100
mls or less (28), the approach using the polyvinylpyr-
rolidone coprecipitate apparently was not found suitable for intravenous use. Therefore it was necessary
to pursue other means of solubilizing acronycine.

The solubility of acronycine in a variety of simple and mixed solvent systems was determined (29) as
shown in Table III. From such data it was obvious that

Table III - Approximate Apparent Solubility of Acrony-
           cine in Various Solvents at about 25° (29)

Solvent	Solubility (mg/ml)
chloroform	275
water	0.002
benzene	40
acetone	32
25% (v/v) acetone in water	20
40% (v/v) propylene glycol in water	8

the solubility problem was not one which could be
solved by using mixed solvent systems which would be
suitable for intravenous purposes. The solubility data
together with the relatively non-polar structural features of the molecule and its rather inconspicuous
melting behavior (m.p. 175-7° (26)) suggested that the
low aqueous solubility was primarily due to a lack of
hydrophilic character rather than to strong intercrys-
talline interactions. Therefore it appeared, as in

Case II above, that the solubility could most readily be increased by decreasing the activity of the dissolved solute molecules. Since it was desired to increase the apparent solubility of acronycine from a value of about 2 mg per liter up to 1 to 2 mg per ml, which represents a 500 to 1000 fold increase, complexation was ruled out due to the much smaller increases normally obtained by that method.

    The solubility of acronycine in acidic solution is shown in Fig. 4 and it was obvious that in order to ob-

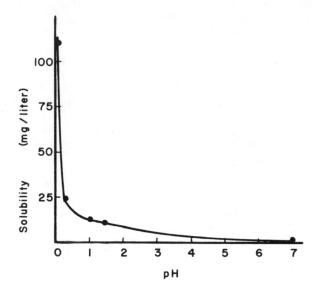

*Figure 4.   The apparent aqueous solubility of acronycine
as a function of pH at 25° (29)*

tain the desired solubility the solution would have to be at pH less than zero, which is impractical. However, the data in Fig. 5 did demonstrate that through the introduction of a charge on the acronycine molecule

it was possible to greatly increase apparent solubility. The problem then was one of introducing and maintaining such a charge in a medium compatible with the
physiological state.

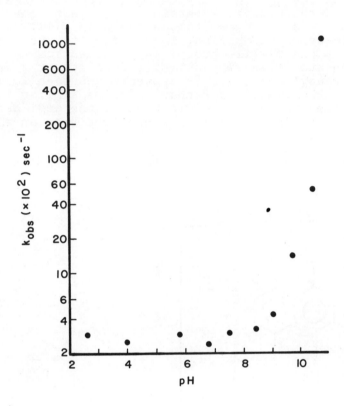

*Figure 5. Plot showing the effects of pH on the observed
first order rate constant for the hydrolysis of the acetylacronycinium ion at 25°. The data points were obtained in a variety
of aqueous buffers at an ionic strength of unity (29, 30).*

One method of achieving this goal was through the
preparation of a derivative which possessed electrolyte
properties. But, the major drawback in this case, as
in Case II, was the absence of chemical sites which
would lend themselves to the formation of derivatives
which would readily and rapidly release free acronycine
following intravenous administration.

An inspection of the acid-base chemistry of acronycine and related compounds (29) ultimately provided
the solution to the problem of the lack of useful sites
suitable for preparing a chemically derived pro-drug.
It appeared that the protonation of acronycine actually
occurs at the carbonyl oxygen which results in aromati-
zation of the nitrogen-containing ring with quaternati-
zation of the nitrogen atom as shown in VIII. This
cationic species contains, in addition to the positive
charge, a phenol-like group. Replacement of the acidic
hydrogen atom with a less labile substituent such as an
alkyl or acyl group was an apparent approach for maintaining an aromatic quaternary species similar to VIII.
For the reasons discussed in Case I, the acyl derivative (IX) again seemed more attractive than an alkyl
derivative.
      The first derivative synthesized, acetylacronyci-
nium (IXa) perchlorate, was prepared by heating acrony-

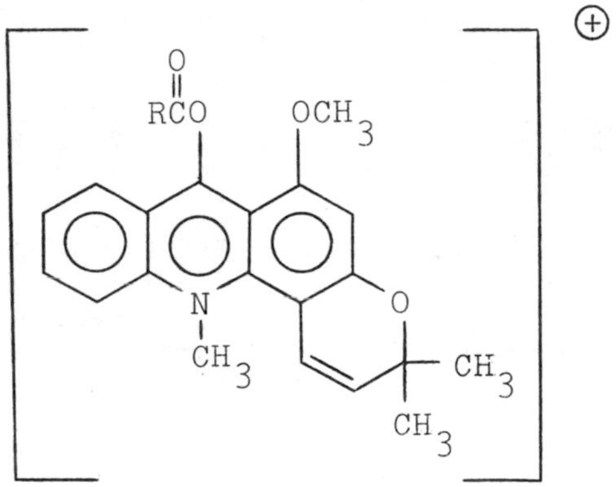

IX a, R = -CH$_3$

IX b, R = -CH$_2$CH$_3$

IX c, R = -CH(CH$_3$)$_2$

IX d, R = -C(CH$_3$)$_3$

IX

Acylacronycinium Ion

cinium perchlorate in acetic anhydride (29). The salt
obtained was found to hydrolyze rather rapidly in aqueous solution to yield acronycine. Because of such hydrolysis only approximate values of the solubility of
the salt could be obtained, but it appeared that the
solubility increase obtained was greater than 100 fold.
Since the apparent solubility of the acetylacronycinium

ion would be expected to be dependent upon the nature of the anion in the salt, a number of different salts were prepared and their approximate aqueous solubilities are given in Table IV. From this data alone it appeared that phosphate or chloride salts might be the most useful because of their high solubilities but it was found that all but the perchlorate salt were extremely difficult to prepare and underwent rather rapid decomposition in the solid state. Thus despite its lower solubility the acetylacronycinium perchlorate salt was the substance which was chosen for more detailed study (29).

Table IV - Approximate Aqueous Solubility of Various Acetylacronycine Salts at Room Temperature (29).

acetylacronycine salt	solubility $(mg/ml)^a$
perchlorate	$\sim$ .25
sulfate	$\sim$ 1.5
phosphate	$\sim$12
bromide	$\sim$ 6
chloride	$\sim$12

a Concentrations are expressed in terms of acronycine in the solution.

The reaction of acetylacronycinium perchlorate in water and aqueous buffer was studied and it was found that the regeneration of acronycine from the acetylacronycinium ion was quantitative (29). Kinetic studies demonstrated that the rate of hydrolysis of the ester linkage was essentially independent of both pH and buffer concentration over a range of pH 0-7. However, at pH greater than 8, hydroxide catalysis was observed. Some of the kinetic data obtained (29) is shown in Fig. 5 where it can be seen that at 25° the hydrolytic rate at pH values below 8 is about 2.8×10^{-2} minute^{-1} which corresponds to a half-life of about 25 minutes. From studies of the temperature dependence of the hydrolysis reaction (29), it appeared that at a body temperature of 37°, the in vitro half-life for hydrolysis would be only about 5 minutes. Although such rapid hydrolysis is desired following parenteral administration, the overall instability presents problems in the preparation of the intravenous formulation. The difficulty arises from a combination of factors which include the low solubility of acronycine, the high apparent concentration of acronycine (as the acetylacronycinium per-

chlorate) desired, and the rather rapid hydrolysis of
the acetylacronycinium ion. As an illustration of the
problem, consider a solution containing the acetylacronycinium perchlorate at a concentration corresponding
to the equivalent of 0.2 mg of acronycine per ml. Upon
hydrolysis of 5% of the acetylacronycinium salt, which
would occur in only about 2 minutes (at room temperature) a five fold supersaturated solution of acronycine
would result. Moreover, the above example is an optimistic one in that no consideration was given to the
hydrolysis likely to occur during the preparation of
the solution.

In light of the above stability problems, it was
necessary to consider approaches by which the hydrolytic stability of the soluble acetylacronycinium ion
could be increased. In view of the pH-profile (Fig.
5), the stability could not be enhanced by pH adjustment and thus more elaborate approaches had to be considered.

Initially, it was felt that the introduction of a
more bulky acyl group would reduce the rate of hydrolysis through steric effects (15). In order to evaluate
this approach, the perchloride salts of IXb, IXc, and
IXd were prepared and the hydrolysis of each was studied at 25° and pH 7.0 or 7.5. Somewhat surprisingly,
the results showed that the hydrolytic rates for all
four of the acetylacronycinium perchlorate salts were
essentially independent of the nature of the acyl group
and the half-life for all was about 25 minutes. This
apparent complete lack of any dependence of the stability on the structure of the acyl group prompted the
consideration of an alternative method for attaining
greater stability.

Earlier work by Higuchi and associate (31,32,33)
had shown that complex formation between organic species in solution could alter their chemical behavior
such as the susceptibility to hydrolysis. Those results led to the consideration of complexing as a potential method for stabilizing the acetylacronycinium
ion.

For many of the same reasons mentioned in Case II,
gentisic acid was chosen as a potential ligand and its
effects on the stability of acetylacronycinium ion were
studied. Some of the results obtained (29) are shown
in Fig. 6.

The observed decrease in hydrolytic rate which occurs with increasing gentisate concentration can be attributed to the formation of complexes between the gentisate and acetylacronycinium ions. Such complex species appear to decrease the susceptibility of the acet-

ylacronycinium ion to hydrolysis. Studies carried out
in more acidic solutions showed a much lesser enhancement of the acetylacronycinium ion stability by the
gentisic acid species, indicating that the effective
ligand is the gentisate ion (29).

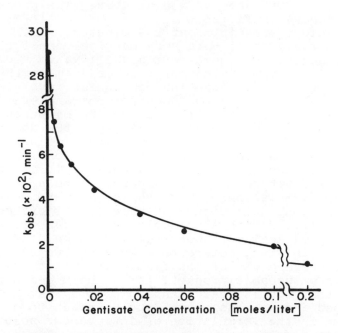

*Figure 6.   Plot of the effects of the gentisate on the observed
first order rate constant for the hydrolysis of the acetylacronycinium ion at 25° (29, 30)*

The non-linear data in Fig. 2 has been shown (29)
to fit a model based on the formation of both 1:1 and
2:1 (gentisate ion: acetylacronycinium ion) complexes.
In both such complexes the hydrolytic stability of the
acetylacronycinium ion was greatly enhanced relative to
the uncomplexed material.

A full and detailed discussion of the model used
in the mathematical treatment of data such as that
shown in Fig. 6 is not essential for the present dis-

cussion and since such information is available elsewhere (<u>29</u>,<u>30</u>), it will be omitted here.
     From the data in Fig. 6 it may be shown that by
adding 0.2 <u>M</u> gentisate ion to the solution described
earlier (containing the equivalent of 0.2 mg of acronycine per ml as the acetylacronycinium perchlorate salt)
hydrolysis of 5% of the acetylacronycinium ion would
only occur after about 45-50 minutes. The production
of a saturated solution, which corresponds to 1% hydrolysis, would result in about 8-9 minutes. Although such
a system would still be a very marginal one for clinical use due to its short-term stability, it represents
a significant improvement over the system in the absence of gentisate. Continuing studies involving the
use of higher gentisate concentrations and evaluation
of other more effective ligands are being pursued.
Also, recent results (<u>34</u>) suggest that the solubility
of free acronycine in aqueous gentisate solution may be
enhanced several fold through complexation. On the basis of the work done and that underway, it is felt that
in the near future it will be possible to prepare a
pro-drug formulation of acronycine, as a reconstitut-
able solution, utilizing a soluble acetylacronycinium
salt stabilized with a suitable ligand such as gentisate. A good deal more work remains to be done, both <u>in</u>
<u>vitro</u> and <u>in vivo</u>, before that goal can be achieved.
However, regardless of the final outcome of this study
in terms of useable product, it has been demonstrated
that rather sophisticated and complex systems may be
developed and used as a pro-drug approach to overcoming
problems in the formulation of intravenous solutions of
cytotoxic agents.

<u>Summary</u>

     The above cases represent some of the more suc-
cessful applications of the pro-drug approach to overcoming problems encountered in the intravenous delivery
of cytotoxic agents. It should be obvious that the development of suitable pro-drugs involves a good deal
more than simply preparing some new chemical species.
There must be a rationale for choosing the new species
and the total system must be reversible under biological conditions in order to achieve any degree of success. Whether or not any of the pro-drug systems discussed ever becomes medically important is largely dependent upon the biological properties inherent in the
parent drug itself. Therefore, while the approaches
illustrated here in the cases of cytotoxic agents may
not prove to be important in these particular systems

they may ultimately be extrapolated to other systems involving other promising drugs.

It has been this author's objective in the above cases to discuss and review the rationale which was involved in the development and evaluation of the approaches used and not to delve into the details of these studies which are or will be reported elsewhere as indicated in the literature citations and especially references (8)(23)(29) and (30).

Acknowledgements

The author wishes to recognize the partial support of this work by contract #N01-CM-23217 from the Division of Cancer Treatment, National Cancer Institute, National Institute of Health, Department of Health, Education and Welfare. In addition, special thanks are extended to those persons who were responsible for much of the work which has been reviewed here. A list of these persons includes D. W. A. Bourne, T. Higuchi, C-H. Huang, B. Krielgard, B. J. Rawson, R. D. Shaffer, K. B. Sloan and W. Waugh.

Literature Cited

1. Benet, L. Z., in "Drug Design", E. J. Ariens, ed., Vol. IV, pp. 9-11, Academic Press, New York, 1973.
2. Wagner, J. G., "Biopharmaceutics and Relevant Pharmacokinetics", pp. 61-2, Drug Intelligence Publications, Hamilton, Ill., 1971.
3. Hess, B., "Enzymes in Blood Plasma", pp. 7-18, Academic Press, New York, 1963.
4. Beck, M. T., "Chemistry of Complex Equilibria", pp. 21-3, Van Nostrand Reinhold Co., London, 1970.
5. Medical News, JAMA (1974), 230, 189.
6. LePage, G. A., Advances in Enzyme Regulation (1970), 8, 323.
7. Cohen, S. S., Prog. in Nucleic Acid Res. Mol. Biol. (1966), 5, 1.
8. Repta, A. J., Rawson, B. J., Shaffer, R. D., Sloan, K. B., Bodor, N., and Higuchi, T., J. Pharm. Sci. (1975), 64, 392.
9. Davignon, J., and Cradock, J. (of the National Cancer Institute) personal communications, Aug., 1972.
10. Bloch, A., Robins, M. J., and McCarthy, J. R., Jr., J. Med. Chem. (1967), 10, 908.
11. Koshima, R., and LePage, G. A., Cancer Res. (1968) 28, 1014.

12. White, F. (of the National Cancer Institute, per-
     sonal communication, May, 1973.
13. Wheeler, L. M. (of Parke, Davis and Co.) personal
     communication, Aug., 1972.
14. Rawson, B. J., Unpublished data (from this labora-
     tory).
15. March, J., "Advanced Organic Chemistry; Reactions,
     Mechanisms and Structures", pp. 233-245, McGraw-
     Hill, New York, 1968.
16. Blum, R. H., Livingston, R. B., and Carter, S. K.,
     Europ. J. Cancer (1973), 9, 195.
17. Takita, H. and Didolkar, M. S., Cancer Chemother.
     Rep. (1974), 58, 371.
18. Cradock, J. (of the National Cancer Institute)
     personal communication, Oct., 1973.
19. National Cancer Institute, Progress reports from
     the Warner-Lambert Research Institute (Contract
     #72-3250), Aug., 1972.
20. "Toxic Substances List", p. 472 (1973), U. S. De-
     partment of Health, Education and Welfare, Rock-
     ville, Maryland, 1973.
21. "Merck Index", 85th Ed., p. 486, P. G. Stecher,
     ed., Merck and Co., Rahway, New Jersey, 1968.
22. Higuchi, T. and Pitman, I. H., J. Pharm. Sci.
     (1973), 62, 55.
23. Krielgård, B., Higuchi, T., and Repta, A. J.,
     (Manuscript submitted to J. Pharm. Sci., January,
     1975).
24. Higuchi, T. and Connors, K. A., "Advances in Ana-
     lytical Chemistry and Instrumentation", Vol. IV,
     pp. 128-193, C. N. Reilly, ed., Interscience, New
     York, 1965.
25. Svoboda, G. H., Poore, G. A., Simpson, P. J., and
     Bodor, G. B., J. Pharm. Sci. (1966), 55, 758.
26. C. A. Hewitt, Stanford Research Institute reports
     to the National Cancer Institute, Nos. 758 and 770
     1968.
27. Svoboda, G. H., Sweeney, M. J., and Walking, W.
     D., J. Pharm. Sci. (1971), 60, 333.
28. Davignon, J. P. (of the National Cancer Institute)
     personal communication, March, 1972.
29. Bourne, D. W. A., Doctoral Dissertation, Univer-
     sity of Kansas, 1974.
30. Bourne, D. W. A., Higuchi, T., and Repta, A. J.,
     A presentation to the Basic Pharmaceutical Section
     of the Academy of Pharmaceutical Sciences, Fall
     meeting, 1973, San Diego. Detailed manuscripts on
     the work have been submitted for publication to J.
     Pharm. Sci. and may be expected to appear in print
     in late 1975.

31. Higuchi, T. and Lachman, L., J. Pharm. Sci. (1955) 44, 521.
32. Lachman, L. and Higuchi, T., ibid. (1957), 46, 32.
33. Lachman, L., Ravin, L., and Higuchi, T., ibid. (1956), 45, 290.
34. Huang, C.-H., Master's Dissertation, University of Kansas, 1975.

6

The Effect of a Pro-drug of Epinephrine (Dipivalyl Epinephrine) in Glaucoma—General Pharmacology, Toxicology, and Clinical Experience

DAVID A. McCLURE

Allergan Pharmaceuticals, Irvine, Calif. 92664

Epinephrine has been used for many years in the treatment of the condition called glaucoma. Glaucoma is a disease where the pressure within the eye increases to a point where damage to the visual apparatus occurs and, if left unchecked, could lead to a significant deminuation in visual acuity and eventually, blindness.

The reasons for this pressure increase are numerous and we will touch on these shortly. However, first, let us examine the anatomy of the eye and how glaucoma comes about. Figure 1 shows a cross section of an eye. From the crystalline lens backward is one chamber filled with a thick, viscus fluid that does not move. Another chamber, that is in front of the lens and the Zonule ligament, is actually composed of two chambers with fluid circulating between. This fluid is called the aqueous humor. The path of the aqueous humor is from the ciliary body, through the pupil, and out the trabecular meshwork and an area called the Canal of Schlemm. Figure 2 is a close-up of the area of fluid circulation and drainage.

Now, we mentioned earlier that glaucoma results from an increase in the intraocular pressure (IOP). The normal IOP averages around 17 mmHg. This pressure can increase in 3 ways: 1) a greater influx of fluid into the envelope of the eye while maintaining a constant outflow, 2) a decreased outflow while maintaining a constant inflow or, 3) a combination of the two. We are concerned primarily (in simple primary glaucoma) with a decrease in the outflow of aqueous fluid. Now what happens if the IOP goes up 10 to 20 mmHg from normal and is maintained at that level? In

other words, why is glaucoma bad? The pressure that
is built up in the front part of the eye is reflected
to the back part of the eye where, of course, the
most vital parts of the eye reside. Figure 3 is a
photograph of the retina. This is the point where
the optic nerve and blood vessels emerge. As the
pressure increases, the disc containing the nerve
and blood vessels is pushed back and a condition
called cupping occurs. This results in a decreased
visual field (peripheral) and as the condition con-
tinues, vision gets worse.

The main adrenergic compound used today is
Chronic simple glaucoma has been treated both
medically and surgically. Medically, there are a
variety of drugs currently available. These are
primarily cholinergic agents such as pilocarpine and
adrenergic agents such as epinephrine. There are
pros and cons for the use of each group. For example,
the cholinergics cause miosis (i.e., a small pupil)
and enough accomodative spasm (i.e., decreased ability
to focus) that reading is difficult, driving at night
is difficult, etc. In addition, because some cholinergics do not penetrate into the eye very well, the
frequency of administration is at an inconvenient,
6 to 8 times per day. In addition, because most of
the cholinergics are esters or lactones, the high
level of local esterase enzymes requires the increased
frequency of administration. Even with all these
inconveniences, miotics are used extensively and tend
to work quite well. Their mechanism of action is
probably vasodilation which permits a greater exit
of aqueous fluid from Schlemm's Canal.

The main adrenergic compound used today is
epinephrine. This compound appears to have a twofold
effect on the maintenance of IOP. The first is the
beta adrenergic mechanism which, similar to the
cholinergic agents, opens up the episcleral blood
vessels permitting a greater fluid loss from the
canal of Schlemm. This appears to be brought about
by the stimulation of epinephrine on the beta adrenergic receptors in episcleral blood vessels and also
those residing in the Canal of Schlemm and perhaps
even in the trabecular meshwork. In addition,
epinephrine has a vasoconstrictive mechanism, i.e.,
the alpha adrenergic mechanism, which may act by
decreasing the production of aqueous fluid from the
ciliary body.

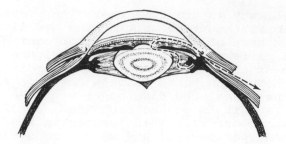

Figure 1

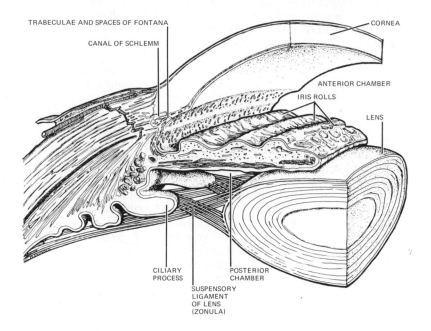

TRABECULAE AND SPACES OF FONTANA

CANAL OF SCHLEMM

CORNEA

ANTERIOR CHAMBER

IRIS ROLLS

LENS

CILIARY PROCESS

SUSPENSORY LIGAMENT OF LENS (ZONULA)

POSTERIOR CHAMBER

Figure 2

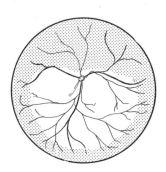

Figure 3

Even though epinephrine appears to have this unique twofold mechanism of action, a number of problems arise, like the cholinergics, with its use. Table 1 illustrates some of these problems.

Table 1

Problems of Epinephrine use in Glaucoma

I.   Duration of Action
 	
II. Side Effects
     A. Ocular
     B. Systemic
 	
III. Bioavailability
 	
IV. Stability

Duration of action. When administered intravenously, the cardiovascular, pulmonary and other effects from epinephrine are over within 10 minutes. When instilled into the eye, a dilated pupil occurs in 10 to 15 minutes and the dilation lasts up to an hour. The duration of lowering of IOP from epinephrine can be seen in Figure 4. The concentration of epinephrine (2%) used in these data represents the highest concentration available. It is presented here to demonstrate the peak activity time of 4 hours and a duration of action of between 12 and 24 hours. The metabolic pathways for epinephrine can be seen in Figure 5.

The side effects occurring from epinephrine topically applied to the eye are both local ocular side effects and systemic. Table 2 illustrates some of these effects.

To get around all these problems with epinephrine, we were fortunate to get a chance to examine an analogue of epinephrine and possibly what is felt to be a pro-drug of epinephrine. Figure 6 shows the chemical structure of epinephrine and its pro-drug, dipivalyl epinephrine (DPE).

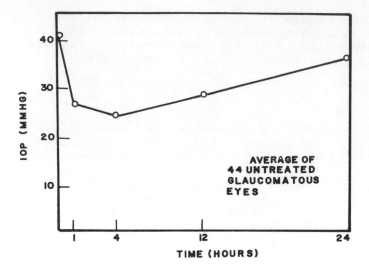

Archives of Ophthalmology

Figure 4.   Response to 1 drop 2% epinephrine (1)

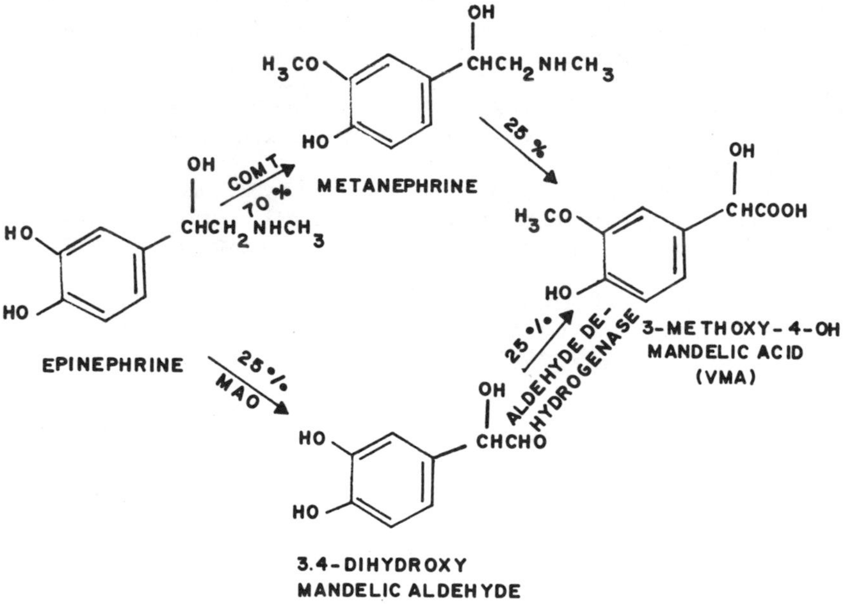

Figure 5

Table 2

Ocular Side Effects of Topical Epinephrine	
I. Hyperemia	V. Browache
II. Mydriasis (Photophobia)	VI. Adrenochrome Deposits
III. Corneal Edema	VII. Tolerance
IV. Allergic Sensitivity	VIII. Maculaopathy

Systemic Side Effects of Topical Epinephrine

  I. Cardiovascular
     A. Cardiac Arrhythmias
     B. Blood Pressure Elevation
     C. Cerebrovascular Accidents

 II. Pallor, Dizziness, Tremor

III. Fear, Anxiety, Tenseness, Restlessness

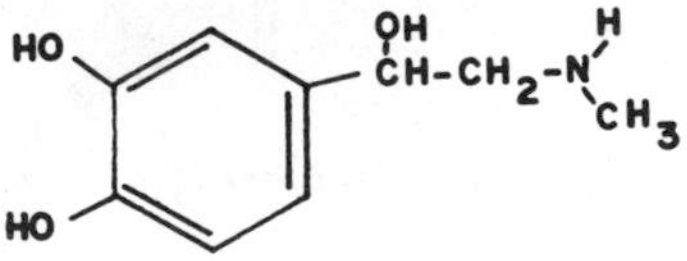

EPINEPHRINE (Mol. Wt. 183.20)

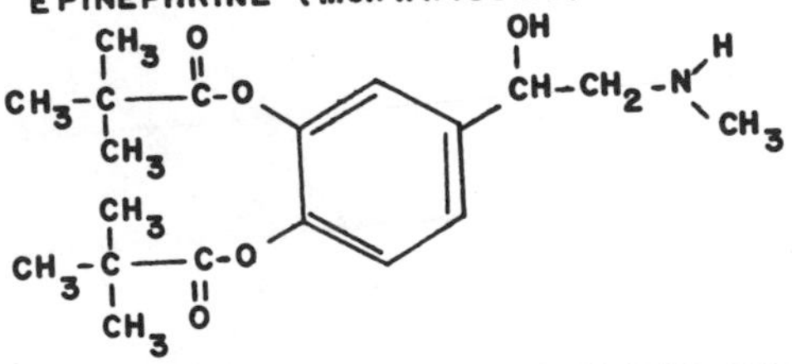

DIPIVALYL EPINEPHRINE (DPE, Mol. Wt. 387.904)

Figure 6

Table 3

	Proposed Advantages of DPE
I.	Increased Duration of Action
II.	Increased Bioavailability
III.	Increased Potency
IV.	Decreased Side Effects
V.	Increased Stability

Table 3 shows the proposed advantages of DPE over epinephrine.

Why an increased duration of action with DPE? Figure 7 illustrates the possible reason for an increased duration of action. The main metabolic pathway of epinephrine is via an enzyme called catechol-o-methyl transferase (COMT). This enzyme methylates the meta hydroxyl in epinephrine. This hydroxyl, as well as the para hydroxyl are not free in DPE. The pivalyl moities are probably slowly removed by local esterase enzymes so that COMT can then act. This would take a prolonged period of time, thus causing a "sustained release" epinephrine.

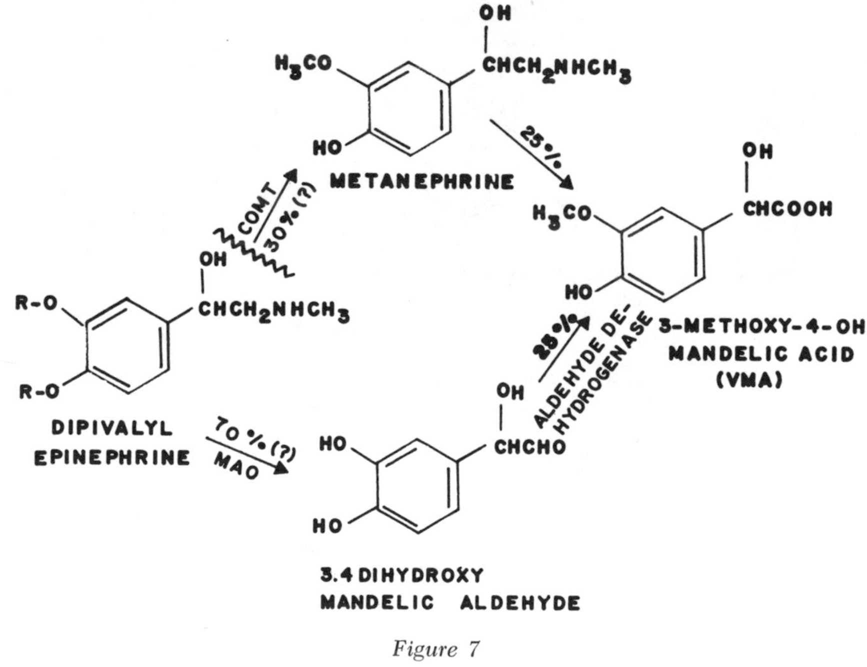

Figure 7

Why an increased bioavailability? It is very
evident that DPE is much more lipophilic than epinephrine by virtue of the two large pivalyl groups at-
tached to the two hydroxyls of epinephrine. In addition, DPE maintains a high degree of hydrophilicity.
Therefore, by its dual solubilities, it fits in very
nicely to the present day absorption theories. The
cornea of the eye is the barrier drugs must overcome
in order to be absorbed into the eye. The cornea is
composed of three layers: an epithelium and an endothelium, both of which require drugs to be lipophilic
if they are to be absorbed and, the stroma; sand-
wiched between the epithelium and endothelium that
required a drug to be hydrophilic for penetrability.
By the dual solubility of DPE, its penetrability into
the eye is greater than the less lipophilic epinephrine molecule.

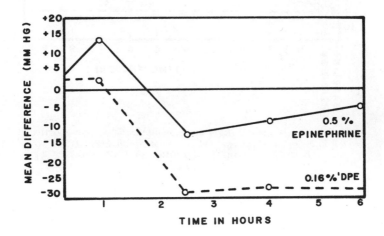

Figure 8.   Comparison of IOP effects in rabbits

Why an increased potency? If more material gains
access to the inside of the eye it will then, on a
relative basis, be more potent. Figure 8 shows a
comparison between 0.5% epinephrine and 0.16% DPE
DPE on the IOP of unanesthetized rabbits. The effects

are obvious. Figure 9 illustrates a dose-response of
DPE on causing pupillary dilation.

On the differential side effect studies, a
comparison of DPE to epinephrine relative to blood

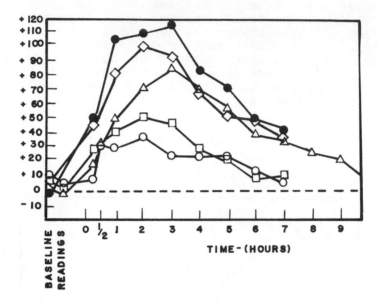

*Figure 9. Mean percent differences in mydriatic response between
treated eyes and control eyes when treated with DPE: 0.20% (○),
0.25% (□), 0.30% (△), 0.40% (◇), 1.00% (●)*

pressure and heart rate effects after intravenous
administration was carried out in dogs and cats.

Figures 10 and 11 compare the effects of intravenously administered DPE and epinephrine on the
blood pressure and heart rate in anesthetized dogs.
It is evident that DPE has significantly less effect
on blood pressure and heart rate than epinephrine.
In a similar fashion, the effect of DPE and epinephrine on the blood pressure of anesthetized atropi-
nized cats may be seen in Figure 12.

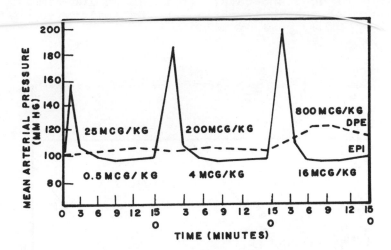

Figure 10. *Effect of I.V. epinephrine and DPE on blood pressure in dogs*

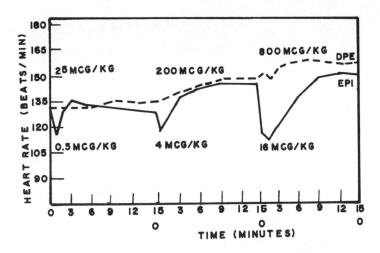

Figure 11. *Effect of I.V. epinephrine and DPE on heart rate in dogs*

DPE is, then, about 100 to 400 times weaker
than epinephrine in affecting the cardiovascular
systems of dogs and cats.   It is about 100 times
more potent than epinephrine in its ability to lower
IOP.

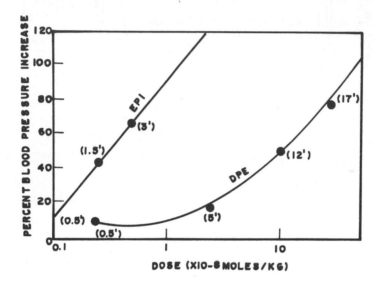

Figure 12.   The effect of epinephrine and DPE on the arterial blood
              pressure of the anesthetized atropinized cat

Finally, the effect of DPE on humans with
glaucoma may be seen in Figure 13.   It can be seen
that the response elicited by DPE is pronounced.   If
one subtracts the contralateral control eye (normal
diurnal response) from the treated eye, it can be
see that DPE produced a marked reduction in IOP.

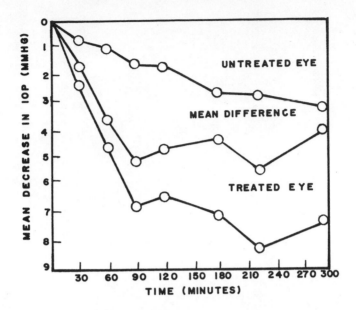

Figure 13. The mean effect of one drop of 0.025% DPE on the IOP of nine glaucomatous individuals.

Summary

    The dipivalyl analogue of epinephrine has been shown to produce fewer side effects and greater potency than the parent compound. These results have been found in both animal and human studies. More studies are to be carried out which will amplify these data and perhaps lead to a better understanding of the mechanism of action of this epinephrine pro-drug.

Literature Cited

    1. L. L. Garner, W. W. Johnstone, E. J. Ballintine, M. E. Carroll, Arch Opth. (1959), 62, 230.

INDEX

INDEX